THE
RIPPLE
EFFECT

THE
RIPPLE
EFFECT

HOW BETTER SEX CAN
LEAD TO A BETTER LIFE

DR. GAIL SALTZ

RODALE

Sex and Values at Rodale
We believe that an active and healthy sex life, based on mutual consent and respect between partners, is an important component of physical and mental well-being. We also respect that sex is a private matter and that each person has a different opinion of what sexual practices or levels of discourse are appropriate. Rodale is committed to offering responsible, practical advice about sexual matters, supported by accredited professionals and legitimate scientific research. Our goal—for sex and all other topics—is to publish information that empowers people's lives.

Rodale books may be purchased for business or promotional use or for special sales. For information, please write to: Special Markets Department, Rodale Inc., 733 Third Avenue, New York, NY 10017

Printed in the United States of America
Rodale Inc. makes every effort to use acid-free ∞, recycled paper ♻.

Book design by Judith Abbate
Illustrations © The New Yorker Collection 2008 from cartoonbank.com.
All Rights Reserved.

Library of Congress Cataloging-in-Publication Data
Saltz, Gail.
    The ripple effect : how better sex can lead to a better life / Gail Saltz.
        p.   cm.
    ISBN-13 978–1–60529–877–1 hardcover
    ISBN-10 1–60529–877–8 hardcover
    1. Women.   2. Sex.   3. Identity (Psychology)   4. Women—Sexual behavior.
I. Title.
HQ46.S3334   2009
155.6'33—dc22   2008042322

Distributed to the trade by Macmillan

2   4   6   8   10   9   7   5   3   1   hardcover

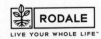

To Lenny, my love

CONTENTS

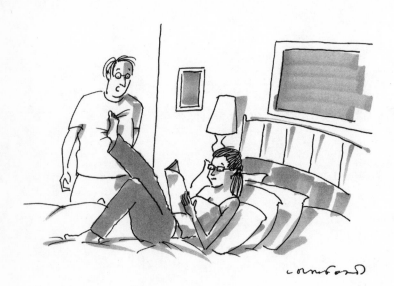

"*I assume that's a no?*"

INTRODUCTION

I am a therapist. Over the years I have seen several hundred women in my practice in New York City. As the psychiatrist on the *Today* show, I have had many others write to me with their concerns. Some women are depressed because they are dangerously in debt. Maybe their husbands aren't working, and they can't make ends meet with just one salary. In other cases, women make more money than their boyfriends or husbands and are afraid of upsetting the balance of power in their relationships. Some women come to me because their children are having trouble at school and they blame themselves. Some have found themselves taking care of an aging parent and reliving old resentments. Some are afraid of failing in their careers; still others are afraid of succeeding. Often a woman starts by describing a small voice in her head, a nagging feeling that something isn't right, that something is missing. With the women I see in my practice, we talk. We go back and forth, discussing not only what's on their minds that day but also what hopes, fears, or regrets they may have held on to for years. Eventually, when we get to the root of the problem, almost always it's sex.

Aristotle said, *Know yourself.* I agree, but when I think about how to advise women patients—and 9 out of 10 patients of mine during the course of my 15 years of practice have been women—I add one key word: *Know your sexual self.*

Women have far more to feel great about than most of us realize. As a woman, you carry within yourself the source of life. It is a well of power that you are born with, and women who understand that power—who understand themselves sexually—live life more fully, no matter their occupations or their marital or parental status. We've all seen the sort of woman who can walk into a room and *pow!* Everybody feels a pull toward her, a great gravitational tug. She has a *presence.* She might not be supermodel "beautiful" or have an hourglass figure. She hasn't necessarily spent more time at the gym than any other woman in the room, or had breast implants or Botox. What she has is something special that radiates from within. She's confident. She's dynamic. She's comfortable in her skin. You can see it in how she holds herself and how she behaves. You look at her, and you think, "She's got it going on."

My goal is to help you become that kind of woman.

In this book I'm going to introduce you to a new approach to your sexuality, one that will help you connect or reconnect with your sexual self. I won't be counseling you to lift a leg here or shift a hip there. Self-help shelves in bookstores are already overburdened with claims that you can improve your sex life by inserting tab A into slot B while holding button C. That approach might help you feel good physically during sex, but it doesn't get at your deeper sexual self. Seeing sex only in physical terms is an old-fashioned and ineffective approach that is based on a fundamental misunderstanding, like treating tuberculosis with breathing exercises, which we did before we knew that tuberculosis is caused by bacteria. We know better now.

We should know better ways to approach our sexuality, too. I believe we've been going about it the wrong way. We've been working from the outside in, hoping that a physical change will make a lasting difference in how women experience sex emotionally, even though experience has told us again and again that it won't. Instead, in this book, we're going to be working from the inside out. By changing how you experience sex mentally and emotionally, we're going to make a lasting difference not only in how you experience sex physically but also in how you experience life itself. The key to this new approach won't be what you do in bed. It'll be how you feel about what you do in bed and how you feel about your sexual self. But the real change will be in how you feel about *you*.

The key to this new approach to sexuality will be to ask yourself: What do you actually think about when you think about sex?

Maybe you know the saying: The most powerful sexual organ is the one between your ears. I couldn't agree more. How you see yourself sexually reflects how you think, feel, and behave in almost every other aspect of your life. Why? Because sex *is* the rest of your life in miniature. During sex, you're literally naked to the world, even if the world is only one other person (or even if it's just yourself). When you're that exposed, every aspect of who you think you are stands out in stark relief. Whether you like yourself, accept your flaws, forgive yourself easily, feel strong, or can find contentment in the moment will all determine how you experience what happens in the bedroom (or wherever you happen to be when the mood strikes). How you see yourself in life determines how you see yourself in bed, and vice versa.

How you see yourself sexually doesn't just reflect the rest of your life; it affects it profoundly. It determines how you think, feel, and behave in almost every other arena, public or private. As Louann Brizendine says in her book *The Female Brain,* "the clitoris really is the brain below the waist." Your sexuality isn't just the key to finding out who you are; it's the key to figuring out who you can become. Improve how you see yourself sexually, and you will have not only better sex but also a better life.

If there's a "Eureka!" realization I'd want you to have as the result of reading this book, it's the same one that I've seen my patients experience again and again: The secret to sexual satisfaction is confidence, and the secret to confidence is sexual satisfaction. It might seem like a chicken-and-egg situation, but in this case we know which comes first. It's your sexuality.

Can you achieve a life-changing boost to your confidence without exploring your sexuality? I hear this question all the time from my women patients. I also hear, "Not that! I'll fix anything else. But please, not my sex life!" Men are different. It's not just that their genitals are out there in the open; so are their attitudes toward sex. Men will talk to me about sex in the first session, but for women, sex is more internal, both physically and emotionally. In my experience, women don't mind working on their relationships with family, friends, and colleagues. They readily admit that they can't express their emotions to a parent, or that they need to speak out more at work, but when it comes to sex, their defenses are as high as the Himalayas. I've seen women who have waited months before letting slip the little fact that they haven't had sex for years. Patients will talk about feeling depressed or anxious. They'll blame their problems on the boss, the husband, the kids. They'll blame themselves. All of these complaints might be real and all the finger-pointing might be valid, but peel away the layers and at the core lies this confession: Fulfilling sex, or even any sex at all, isn't part of their lives, whether by choice, design, or neglect.

Exercising, making time for friends, and eating right— women who wouldn't dream of neglecting these aspects of their physical and emotional health will nonetheless see a fulfilling sex life as dispensable. They think sex is for the young, the thin, the single woman with great clothes and lots of time to spend at the gym. In a society absolutely obsessed with sex, youth, and perfect bodies, many women have allowed themselves to sit on the sidelines. A fulfilling sex life is *not* dispensable. It is an essential way of nurturing your body and spirit.

Your sexuality is as much in the head as it is in the heart or the vagina, and that's the female power you need to tap—the one in that powerful sex organ between your ears. Sure, you might be able to show confidence on the outside, and maybe you can even make headway on the other problem areas in your life—your guilt over your child's struggles at school, your anger at the arrogant colleague at work—but your confidence will be false and the solutions temporary. Whether you're not having sex at all or having it all the time but not finding it fulfilling or anywhere in between, the bottom line is the same: If you don't address the most vital part of yourself—your actual life force— you're living what amounts to half a life.

Once upon a time, the vagina was a symbol of power. A woman could change the course of history simply by raising her skirt. Ancient writings tell of women exposing their vaginas and turning back armies, calming seas, scaring lions, increasing harvests. Across cultures and throughout history, the vagina has been viewed as a powerful force of nature. Yet the vagina is also a source of mystery. It works its wonders in obscurity, stealthily, as if by magic. Its power is hidden. It is literally out of sight.

The trouble begins when you allow your vagina to be out of mind, too. When the vagina became a source of shame— think of the Western myth of Eve tempting Adam, how she came to bear responsibility for humankind's banishment from Paradise—culture in general and women in particular lost something essential in their identities. A Hollywood starlet deliberately showing off her lack of underwear to the paparazzi is not a role model of sexual independence; instead, she's perpetuating a stereotype of exploitation. If feminine sexuality is perceived as both dangerous and filthy, then the temptation for women is not to celebrate their own sexuality but to regard it as something separate from themselves, or maybe even to ignore it—to accept their vaginas as only passive receptacles, rather than the active organs they really are. The muscles of the human vagina are exquisitely sensitive on their own terms, expanding, contracting, moistening. They're not passive. They're powerful. I want you to know and to feel this power and to experience how it can help transform your life.

This isn't an empty promise. Dopamine, oxytocin, and endorphins, the neurochemicals and hormones released when a woman has an orgasm, produce a powerful chain reaction that makes her feel on top of the world. To climb that mountain, you first need to understand how a woman's mind and body work together. Studies show that even when women are experiencing the physical evidence of sexual arousal, they often don't feel aroused because they don't *think* they're aroused.

In this book, I will help you change what you think about when you think about sex. I will help you reunite your mind with your body. Maybe we can't single-handedly change what the world thinks of female sexuality, but we can change what *we* think of it. What *you* think of it. What you think of *yourself*.

How you think about your sexuality right now is not your fault, but how you continue to think about your sexuality from this day forward *is* your responsibility. In this book, you'll have the chance to learn to bring female sexual power into everything you do by looking closely at the negative thoughts and stories that define your sexual identity and then changing them into positive ones.

I say "stories" because that's how we actually see ourselves—as characters in a lifelong narrative. We all live our lives according to the narratives we've imagined for ourselves. They're so much a part of you that you think they *are* you. You may not even be aware that they're there. Like all stories, they're true only to the extent that the storyteller—in this case, you— is reliable. Sadly, in most cases, when patients eventually ask themselves how reliable they really are, the answer is: not very.

The first thing I'll do in this book is introduce you to other women (composites of patients I've seen in my own practice) with stories similar to your own. You'll see how they uncovered their damaging stories with my help, and how they discovered the ways those stories affect them in bed and throughout their lives. We'll try to discover what stories define *your* view of your sexual self, where those stories came from, and how to change them.

In particular, we'll look at five types of stories that in my experience we all tell ourselves at one time or another. We'll look at why you might sometimes feel insecure sexually, why you sometimes might feel so guilty that you can't enjoy your sexuality, and why you sometimes feel envious of other people's seemingly perfect sex lives. We'll look at why you sometimes feel more emotionally vulnerable than you actually are and why you sometimes feel more physically vulnerable than you actually are.

We're going to figure out how you can free yourself to be one of the women who are confident. Who know they'll be able to live their lives fully, because they know who they are. Who *like* who they are, are comfortable in their skin, and don't need to turn to anyone else to make them feel whole. Who know their vaginas inside out (pun emphatically intended). Who can give to others because they know they'll also be able to give to themselves. Who know what they want and know how to get it, because they know what they want sexually and know how to get it. Women who know that feeling sexy and voluptuous comes not from how they look, but from how they feel about themselves. Who know that bad things will still happen but that they'll be okay, because they have a core identity that is unshakable. Who can put their energies not only into attracting others but also into being attractive to themselves. Who feel truly alive, and who feel it all the time. Who can walk into a room and *pow!*

This is the power of female sexuality, and soon it could be yours.

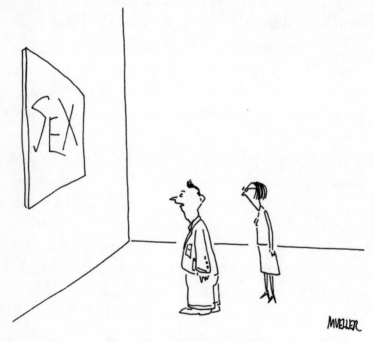

"We could put it in the bedroom."

CHAPTER ONE

THE RIPPLE EFFECT

ALEXANDRA SAID SHE'D COME TO ME because of a quiz in a women's magazine. "I know this sounds ridiculous," she said, "but I was in the pediatrician's waiting room, and there was a copy of some magazine, and I took a quiz in it called 'How Satisfied Are You?'"

She paused, waiting for me to ask the obvious question.

"So," I said, "how satisfied are you?"

"Apparently not very," she said. "My score was a 65. The high end of 'Average.' Not even the low end of 'Above Average.'" She smiled self-deprecatingly. "You'd think they might at least grade on a curve."

"Do you really think a quiz in a magazine can reveal your overall emotional state?" I asked.

"No," she said. "That's not what bothered me."

"So what did bother you?"

"I think the quiz was right. Just sitting there, taking a magazine quiz in a pediatrician's waiting room, I really felt average. Mediocre."

"Why don't you tell me some more details about yourself," I suggested. "Forget for the moment about whether or not you really are 'satisfied' or 'average.' Just tell me what's been going on in your life."

Over the coming weeks, that's just what Alexandra did. She described herself as "just this side of 40," a "workaholic" who actually loves what she's addicted to. She met her husband in a business course in college. Tom, like Alexandra, was a conscientious, success-oriented person who was happier talking about work than anything else. At the beginning of their relationship, she and Tom were a team in every way. Sometimes they would sit up in bed with a notebook open, brainstorming ideas for the small business they hoped to start one day. In the end all their hard work paid off. They got their business off the ground a few years after college, and it was successful. When the time came for them to think about starting a family, she figured they would just transfer their teamwork approach to that part of their life. Raising a child wouldn't be all that big a leap.

It wasn't, for Tom. As Alexandra told me, "He's basically able to take anything new that comes along and simply fold it into his life. A 7-pound screaming infant in the house? No problem!"

Right from the start *she* was overwhelmed. Alexandra was a perfectionist, used to controlling her world, but Caleb was a screaming, colicky mess in her otherwise well-ordered life. No matter what she did, she just couldn't seem to soothe him. For perhaps the first time in her life, Alexandra felt inadequate. That, she told me, is when she first noticed a change in herself. She had become, she said, "moody." Caleb had eventually stopped crying, but he had never stopped being what his pediatrician, his nursery school teacher and her friends called a "high-needs child"—intense, emotional, inflexible, and prone to wild swings of temper that left Alexandra confused about what to do and worried that she might never figure it out. Her "moodiness," she said, persisted to this day. Perhaps worst of all, it was a change that Tom had never noticed.

That's when Alexandra finally got around to talking to me about her sex life. The subject had been curiously absent from our conversations, but it was an absence that I found to be all too common in my practice. Women patients often wait as long as they can before they get around to discussing their sex lives—and the longer they wait, the more important it turns out to be.

In Alexandra's case, Tom's obliviousness to her change in mood became clear to her in bed. Practically every night when work was over and they'd tucked Caleb in, Tom would basically "leap" on her. "He's a guy," she figured. "It's in his blood."

Meaning: It wasn't in *her* blood. Alexandra had told herself that her decreasing interest in sex was "an aging thing," that desire goes down over the course of a marriage, and couples become best friends more than fiery lovers. They had the best marriage among their friends—everybody said so—and that was enough for her. Sometimes it seemed to be enough for

Tom, too. If he collapsed with a beer in front of *SportsCenter* instead of wanting to have sex, she found herself relieved and thinking to herself: "Whew—now I don't have to pretend tonight."

Alexandra didn't want to have to pretend, ever. When she thought back to the days when their lovemaking was long and robust and they seemed sexually indefatigable, when they were a "team" and open with each other about everything, she felt a pang of regret, and not a little guilt at having to deceive Tom now. One night when Tom curled up beside her in bed and planted a hand on her breast, she heard herself say, "We're not 22 anymore, in case you hadn't noticed."

He seemed wounded, not surprisingly. "I don't understand," he said. "Aren't you attracted to me, Alexandra?"

"Of course," she said. Maybe it was pity that motivated her, or guilt at having been so blunt and hurtful, but she began to backtrack. She said that all she meant was that they ought to be more realistic about what they expect from a marriage at this point in time. In her heart of hearts, she knew she had lashed out on purpose. Tom was able to roll with the ways Caleb had changed their lives, and he was better for it. He loved being a dad. She, on the other hand, had just never gotten her footing. She feared she was failing at everything: motherhood, career, and marriage. She felt guilty for not being able to accept Caleb for who he was, and at the same time she resented her son for taking her away from the work and the marriage that had sustained her for so many years. Tom said that he'd try to be more sensitive, and then they had sex.

Afterward, when Tom was asleep, Alexandra lay in the darkness of the bed where they once made long to-do lists after a
vigorous bout of lovemaking, and she thought about how she
now had everything she wanted back then: a great husband, a
beautiful child, a terrific career. She knew she couldn't fully
enjoy her good fortune—not as long as the only way she was
going to score 100 on a magazine quiz was if the subject was
"How Fake Are You?"

ALEXANDRA'S SITUATION WAS MORE COMMON
than you might imagine. Many women have come to see me
because their partners want sex and they don't. Of course,
Alexandra didn't think that was the reason she came to see me,
but that information about her sex life turned out to be the key
to our understanding of her whole life: of who she was, and
who she could become.

Where does your sexual identity come from? How does it
affect your life? These questions are crucial to understanding
the woman you are, and understanding the woman you are is
crucial to finding out how you can change into the woman you
want to be. A powerful woman. A confident woman. A woman
who would be able to score "Extremely" on a "How Satisfied
Are You?" pop quiz.

Throughout this book we'll be looking at five ways women
like you and me think of ourselves during sex, and how our
sexual identities influence every other part of our lives. I call it
"the ripple effect." Unlike Vegas, what happens in bed doesn't

stay in bed. It emanates outward, in every direction, until it reaches the farthest shores of family, friendships, and work. It's always there; it's always everywhere. Touch the surface of your life and you'll feel it. Alexandra took a quiz in a magazine and felt it—and didn't like what she felt.

The ripple effect can be a negative force, but it can also be a positive force. If your sexual identity is vital and powerful, then you'll feel that vitality and power throughout your life—a sense of control, of ownership, of confidence in who you are.

Some of this ripple effect is physical. You can think of sex as a chemical cocktail, since a number of hormones are released after sex and have beneficial effects. Oxytocin causes relaxation and feelings of love and bonding. Endorphins are the body's natural painkillers. Immunoglobulin A can help fight off colds. Many people find that after sex they fall asleep easily, and getting a good night's sleep has many health benefits.

You can think of active sex as an aerobic exercise. It's good for your heart. It tones your stomach, back, and buttock muscles. It relieves stress and—don't laugh—it gives your vagina a healthy workout.

Like other muscles, the vagina is a "use it or lose it" organ. The more you use your pelvic muscles, the more they stay in shape. The less you use them, the more likely they are to atrophy, until sex can actually become painful. (Pelvic muscles also affect bladder control; the better shape those muscles are in, the better your bladder control will be later in life or after having babies. Who wants to pee every time she sneezes or coughs?)

I'm pleased to say that women do seem to be giving their pelvic muscles a greater workout than ever before. According to a study conducted at the Institute of Neuroscience and Physiology at Gothenburg University in Sweden over a period of 30 years, the percentage of married women having sex at age 70 rose from 38 percent in 1971 to 56 percent in 2001. The percentage of women saying that they experienced orgasms during sex also rose dramatically. Probably this change in sexual activity is partly due to improvements in health and fitness, and probably it is partly due to the increasingly tolerant social attitudes toward sex that these seniors learned when they were young. Whatever the reasons, I like to think that these seniors are living proof of a vital lesson—one with a scientific basis: The more sex you have, the more you want to have sex.

Specifically, the more often you have an orgasm, the higher your overall level of sexual desire and arousal. One explanation (shown in small studies) may be that levels of testosterone—the hormone of desire—rise with frequent sexual activity. Which might lead you to ask: Why not just pump women full of testosterone and let 'er rip?

There are two good reasons. Such an approach would certainly increase a woman's desire, but it would also increase the potential for cardiovascular disease, facial hair, and a deep voice, as well as possibly breast cancer and stroke. In the United States testosterone has been deemed too risky in terms of the side effects to make it readily available, though in Europe the testosterone patch was approved in 2007. Some women do have a low testosterone level for their age or menopausal status, and they can indeed get medical help in the United States, but only to raise their testosterone to a normal—and safe—level. Even then the treatment includes increased levels of estrogen to balance the testosterone, since we don't know enough about the side effects of taking testosterone alone.

The second reason doctors wouldn't want to prescribe testosterone for most women is that such a treatment would be beside the point. It wouldn't address the issue that could really make a difference in a woman's life. Unlike men who use Viagra to correct erectile dysfunction or women who have naturally low testosterone levels, most women need to overcome a barrier that is not physical but psychological.

In one recent study, for instance, the sexual medicine group at Vancouver General Hospital in British Columbia found a distinct difference between what happens physically to women undergoing arousal and what they *think* is happening. Objectively, women watching pornography showed body changes signaling arousal—lubrication and bloodflow to the genitals. Subjectively, however, most of the women in the study said they did not feel aroused and were not turned on by the images. For men like Tom—which is to say, for men in general—what is physically happening during arousal and what they think is happening are pretty much the same thing. For women like Alexandra—and for women in general—sexual satisfaction is much more heavily weighted toward the psychological than the physiological. Their bodies may be responding, but their brains aren't.

That's why the medications that researchers have been

studying in the hopes of finding a female equivalent to Viagra would work their wonders by rewiring the brain, not by rerouting bloodflow to the genitals. I believe that even successfully rewiring the female brain would still be missing the point. It would still be a physiological solution. Despite its immediate benefits, it would still be an old-fashioned and ultimately ineffective approach. One that works from the outside in, rather than the inside out; that changes how you experience sex physically, not how you experience sex emotionally; that treats the symptom, not the cause. One that changes *how* you think, not *what* you think.

In this book we're going to do just that. We're going to focus on changing *what* you think about sex. I believe that only when you reunite your physical self with your mental self can you have a chance of becoming a whole self.

I can point to plenty of case histories from my own practice that support this belief. In fact, I'll be pointing to them throughout this book, just as I did with Alexandra and Tom at the beginning of this chapter. I can also point to persuasive medical research. A university group in Portugal, for instance, has been studying the relationship between women's thoughts and behavior during sex for years, and the results have been consistent: Women who have "dysfunctional beliefs" about sex are far more likely to have dysfunctional sex itself—lack of desire or sexual arousal or orgasm. Some examples of these dysfunctional beliefs—negative or nonerotic thoughts—might seem to be of a personal, individual nature: I am sexually incompetent; I am afraid of sex; I think nonmissionary or nonprocreative sex is "wrong." Some might involve body image or age-related issues: Women who are not attractive can't be sexually satisfied; as women age, they get less pleasure from sex; after menopause, women lose their sexual desire altogether. What all these dysfunctional thoughts have in common is that they arise from *stories*—not facts—these women have come to believe. Whether they originated in one woman's upbringing or our common culture, whether they involve one woman's sexuality or female sexuality in general, these stories feel true, but they're not.

A story doesn't have to render you sexually dysfunctional in order to take its toll. We're all at the mercy of the stories we believe about our sexuality. We've all altered our sexual selves to some extent to accommodate these stories. Each of us believes these stories because they feel true, but they're not.

In this chapter we're going to identify the five most common negative stories we all tell ourselves at one time or another about our sexual identities. In later chapters we're going to look at each of these stories in greater detail, we're going to see why they're not true, and we're going to learn to use the power of truth to change them. These aren't stories that necessarily influence you all the time—maybe not even most of the time. You aren't influenced by all five stories at once.

Often enough, individually or in combination, these stories make a difference in what you think about when you think about sex. They determine the thoughts that ripple outward from the bedroom and into the rest of your life. Our job is to change that ripple effect from a negative influence to a positive one.

WHEN YOU THINK
YOU DON'T KNOW WHAT YOU'RE DOING

"A little to the right," you say, and you think, "This is it, this will work," and then it doesn't work, and then you start to wonder whether there's something wrong with you. You think maybe you don't completely understand what your genitals are or how they function. You worry that maybe your genitals don't function.

At some point in your sex life you've probably experienced some form of this self-doubt, if only for a second—which is just long enough to ruin the moment. You might have had a perfectly sound reason for not experiencing sexual pleasure on those occasions: fatigue, distractedness, one glass of wine too many. Or you might not have educated yourself fully about how your genitals work. Whatever the physical facts, a disappointing sexual encounter can leave you feeling emotionally defeated or like a failure in all parts of your life, not just in bed.

Everybody else seems to be functioning well; why aren't you? Is there something wrong with you? What if there is? Do you really want to deal with that? Maybe it's better not to try new things in your life, to explore, to experiment, to broaden your horizons. If you can live without sexual pleasure, then you can live without pleasure, period, right?

Alexandra thought she could. As she and I talked about her husband's, Tom's, boundless sexual energies and her own lack of enthusiasm, we made the unsurprising discovery that Alexandra had begun to question not only her emotional attitude but also her physical abilities. "Maybe it's just hormonal," she said one day. "Maybe I just don't have it in me anymore."

Maybe. Or maybe not. She could have found out; she could have gone to a doctor and gathered hard facts, or she could have lived in ignorance. Alexandra had chosen the latter path, one leading through the landscape of perpetual doubt and denial, without really realizing that she'd made a choice. She was living her life according to the story that she didn't know what she was doing—and that maybe she couldn't even do it.

WHEN YOU THINK
YOU DON'T DESERVE
WHAT YOU HAVE

"A little to the right," you say, and you think, "I'm so demanding," then you wonder what he thinks of you, then you wonder what you think of you. You think maybe "good girls"—happy, clean, and wholesome mommies or wives or older women or young singles—don't lose control. You think you should just shut up and lie there.

Women often wonder how well their sexual partners understand the female anatomy, and they sometimes feel the need to offer advice such as "a little to the right" or "a little to the left" or "faster now." Ideally these requests are part of a healthy give-and-take during sex. Sometimes that give-and-take can take you right out of the moment. It can make you objectify yourself—can make you see a woman and a man having sex. If you like what you see, great! If what you see leaves you feeling a little guilty or ashamed, not so great.

A little guilt goes a long way. You feel like you've done something wrong, so you punish yourself. You deny yourself that dessert because you think you don't deserve it, and you don't deserve that promotion, either, or your husband's love, or your own self-respect. You then feel guilty about punishing yourself, so you punish yourself some more. This can go on and on. At its most extreme, a sense of sexual guilt can leave a woman walking around feeling like a "slut"—and maybe even punishing herself by being one, just to feel worse about herself.

Alexandra didn't feel like a slut. Quite the opposite. In their youth, she and Tom had joyful sex, uninhibited sex during which they freely traded desires and fantasies. If Alexandra stepped out of the moment and saw herself objectively, as a young woman in the middle of having sex, she liked what she saw. By the time in her life that she no longer wanted to have sex but did anyway, she *didn't* like what she saw. She had turned into the antislut.

She knew that Tom's desires were normal, if maybe a little overheated. So she gave in, time and again, being ever the obedient sexual partner because she didn't want to feel guilty or admit to Tom the inadequacy that she felt in the bedroom and in other areas of her life. She just shut up and lay there. She wound up feeling guilty anyway, because she was going through the motions and being dishonest with Tom in precisely the kind of situation where the two of them used to be completely open and honest. And then the one time she didn't give in and instead reminded Tom that they weren't their gymnastic 22-year-old selves anymore, she wounded him, and she ended up feeling even more guilty. She went back to going through the motions and feeling less guilty but guilty nonetheless and trying to figure out with my help at what point in her life she had started believing that she doesn't deserve what she has.

WHEN YOU THINK
YOU WANT WHAT YOU DON'T HAVE

"A little to the right," you say, then you think, "Why doesn't he know that?" If you were a guy, you'd make it your business to know that, and hey, you're a woman and you've made it your business to know what's what with him. This whole sex business? Not fair, but life isn't fair.

We all know this. Still, sometimes the differences between the sexes can seem especially unfair, particularly during sex, when those differences are unmistakable. I'm not saying that the differences are *always* unfair to women. You can't be even with your partner every time you're in bed. You have to take turns. Sometimes the moment is more about him, and sometimes the moment is more about you. Women can often find it difficult to muster sympathy for men. It seems like he's always ready to go. What's *he* got to complain about?

Maybe one time you don't go on to say, "Okay, now just a bit *more* to the right." Maybe next time you don't say anything at all. You let him figure it out. "Go on, big boy, show me what you're made of," and he does—at least as far as he's concerned. As far as you're concerned, though, you've proven that his anatomy is easier. His pleasure is easier. You'll wonder why your pleasure has to be so complicated. You'll look at your partner and think that you're supposed to love him, yet here you are, feeling that maybe he really does have it better than you do.

Even a fleeting appearance of the green-eyed monster in bed can ruin the moment and follow you out of the bedroom and into the streets, where—well, where life just isn't fair. If you already suspect that a lot of people have it better than you do, you'll soon feel that you'll never be even with your friends or colleagues. It's hard to feel satisfied in any area of life when you think that everybody has it better than you.

Alexandra certainly thought life wasn't fair. She'd worked hard, loved hard, and achieved success on her own terms: great husband, great kid, great career. The moment that she started to feel like less than a straight-A adult, when she couldn't calm her son's colic or ease his path in the world, she began to doubt herself. Tom, oblivious, kept plugging away—at life, and at her. He stayed a straight-A businessman, father, and husband. The more he did so, the more she retreated and the more she resented him.

WHEN YOU THINK
YOU'RE EMOTIONALLY VULNERABLE

"A little to the right," you say, then you think, "Oh, great, now he knows," then he actually goes to the right and you know he knows how you work. You begin to wonder what else he knows about how you work. You begin to wonder what else he knows about you.

There's a saying, "Knowledge is power." It's true in life and it's especially true in bed, because sex is all about power. Not necessarily in a negative way. The tangle of bodies, the mixture of pressures, the probing and thrusting and grinding: It's all about physical boundaries, but it can also be about mental boundaries. If you say, "A little to the right," you've ceded some knowledge. Maybe you're scared to let him know what gives you pleasure because you aren't comfortable admitting desires like that. Maybe you're scared to let him know what gives you pleasure because then *he'll* be in control and then he'll have all the power.

Being out of control *can* be scary. In bed as in life, you have your own comfort level as to how much to let go—whether letting go of your physical self while in the throes of passion, or letting go of knowledge of who you are. In general the extent to which you protect yourself from the one person with whom you should be most open and intimate will be an indication of the extent to which you protect yourself from people with whom you have more casual relationships. The extent to which you want to protect yourself can change from one sexual encounter

THE RIPPLE EFFECT 17

to the next, but if the wall you build is too high, it won't just protect you, it will isolate you—from your lover, from your friends and family, from life.

When Alexandra began to feel emotionally vulnerable, she felt she couldn't talk about her fears with Tom, so she shut herself down, both emotionally and physically. Without consciously realizing it, Alexandra had found a way to keep feeling powerful. She knew something important that Tom didn't know; she possessed essential knowledge about herself that he didn't have: She was going through the motions.

The power Alexandra retained was only an illusion. Going through the motions can be a lonely experience, and the more distant she felt from Tom, the more distant she felt from the world. Alexandra might or might not have scored 100 percent on a magazine quiz called "How Fake Are You?," but she definitely would have aced a test titled "Do You Think You're Emotionally Vulnerable?"

WHEN YOU THINK
YOU'RE PHYSICALLY VULNERABLE

"Don't," you say. Not "a little to the right." Not "a little to the left." Just plain old no.

Knowledge is power, but power is power, too. In sex, physical boundaries become a blur and the possibility always exists that one or the other partner might inadvertently go too far. A simple "Ow" is usually enough to reestablish the boundaries (unless the point of the sex play is pain, in which case the partners need to agree beforehand on a set of boundaries that are different but no less inviolable). For women, though, the possibility of physical pain can be daunting. Women and men might potentially be psychological equals; think of women exposing their vaginas to vanquish an invading army. For all I know, you might be physically more dominating than your partner, but on the whole, women and men aren't physical equals, and unlike emotional vulnerability, physical vulnerability for many women isn't just a possibility, it's a reality.

What you do with that reality will define your relationship with your partner. If you come into a relationship already feeling fragile, "to the right" or "to the left" isn't going to matter much. All that will matter is that you don't want that battering ram near you, so you tighten and become rigid. In extreme circumstances you might even lose the ability to believe that sex can ever be pleasurable. The difference between thinking of yourself as emotionally vulnerable and thinking of yourself as physically vulnerable is the difference between feeling guarded and feeling fearful. If your lifelong sense of yourself as fragile is confirmed in the bedroom, with the person you trust most, you can only imagine how fearful you'll feel around people you don't know nearly as well.

Alexandra had never really feared Tom physically, but when she started going through the sexual motions with him, she no longer experienced the once-familiar responses to stimulation:

a pulsing sensation in her veins, a flushing all over, an easing forward, an urging onward, an urging inward. As she said to me, "He gets hard, I stay dry, and in a little while it's over."

"That must be painful," I suggested, and Alexandra nodded quickly. And the anticipation of pain next time, she said, made the situation worse, and therefore the sex more painful. The time after that wound up being even more painful. It was just about then that she told Tom that they weren't 22 anymore. When she told me that, I realized Alexandra had begun to believe the story that she was physically more vulnerable than she actually was.

WE'VE NOW COVERED FIVE COMMON STORIES that keep women from getting the greatest satisfaction out of their sex lives—and out of life, period. You've probably recognized aspects of yourself in most of these stories, if not all of them. Good! That means you're normal, and it gives us a lot to work with. The time has come to find out where these stories come from.

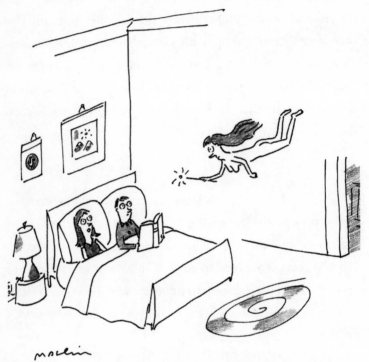

"Owen, look—the good sex fairy."

CHAPTER TWO

HOW YOUR SEXUALITY CAME TO BE

MARIE COULD NOT REMEMBER A SINGLE point in her life when her weight was far from her thoughts. She recalled that when she was a little girl sitting at the dinner table, her mother would slide the butter plate away from her grasp, telling her, "No, Marie, you and I can't have that. It's plain bread and water for us, like two jailbirds!" Her mother would laugh. Marie would pretend to laugh, too, and would then watch enviously as her brother and father took the butter and freely slathered it on their own bread. She and her mother—neither one obese, certainly, but both of them a bit overweight and always struggling to keep those extra pounds off—were like members of a club that no one would want to join: women who perennially had to deny themselves pleasure.

Throughout her life, Marie would remain a part of this club. Her membership was demonstrated frequently at home with her mother: "No offense, honey," her mother told her one night when they sat together in the den letting out the seam in Marie's dress, "but you want to look good, right? You want some boy to go ga-ga over you. When I was your age, I always worried that that would never happen to me. I know you may think your dad isn't exactly a hunk, but believe me, when I met him in college I had to diet like crazy before he would even look at me!"

Then, later on, as 27-year-old Marie flipped through the fashion magazines that arrived in her mailbox each month, she found herself in that same old club, comparing her rounded, too-big body with the long, hipless chopstick figures of the supermodels who graced page after page. All she could think, gazing at those surreally beautiful women, was: "I hate the way I look."

Sometimes, when Marie came home from work at night and sat with a carton of chicken fried rice and a beer, flipping around the TV dial, she would watch a reality show in which women had a chance to change the qualities about themselves that they hated most. Marie fantasized about going on that show and saying to the chic, chilly host, "Get rid of all the blubber! Just take it away; I never want to see it again." She would undergo multiple rounds of liposuction, perfecting her chin, stomach, hips, and thighs, in an attempt to bring her to a place where she could be happy about herself when she looked in the mirror. That, of course, was a fantasy that she could barely imagine. The mirror had always been her enemy. Each time she stood before a plate of reflecting glass, she had to endure a churning wave of shame. Occasionally she even literally flinched when she looked at herself.

She knew, of course, that she was not "morbidly" fat. She wasn't one of those women you don't want to sit next to on an airplane—someone whose body spills over into your seat. She also knew that her body still made her feel depressed and unhappy. The place where she felt it most acutely—perhaps even more acutely than in the cool surface of the mirror—was in the deep and complicated folds of a bed. Whenever Marie went to bed with a man, her negative impressions about her physical self clicked into place, becoming highlighted and exaggerated. As the man touched each part of her body, she imagined it from his point of view. "Now his hand is on my breast," she would think. "He's probably saying to himself: 'It's so big and saggy. I wish she were thin, like that last woman I slept with.' Now he's looking at my stomach. I'd better turn a little into the shadows, so he can't see the rolls of fat there."

She spent so much time during lovemaking thinking about how she looked from the man's perspective that she actually forgot to think about what she felt about the act itself. It was as though she wasn't a person at all, wasn't someone who possessed desires and preferences. Sex became clinical, like having an exam and being found wanting. In a way, it seemed as though sexual pleasure was like a gigantic plate of butter: As Marie reached for it, a hand swept down and firmly pushed it away. Only now, of course, that hand didn't belong to her mother. It belonged to her.

What had prompted Marie to deal with her problem directly was that she became involved in a serious relationship—the first one of her life, she admitted. She loved Philip, she told me. He was funny. He was devoted to her. He even insisted that he liked the way she looked. "He's a little overweight, too," she said, "and he knows it. But for him it's no big deal." For Marie, the deal was getting bigger and bigger. While with other men she had found herself constrained and preoccupied in bed, with Philip she found herself actually becoming phobic. He wasn't critical of her imperfections, but more and more frequently she chose to wear her nightgown when they were together. When he protested, she insisted she was cold. Always, the lights had to be out in the room; the place was as dark as a haunted house. She would turn the lights off; he would turn them back on. They would squabble over this, and invariably she would win.

She recognized that this was a big problem and that it was only getting worse. Lately Philip was starting to pull away. He wasn't happy with how inhibited she was in bed. He thought it was *him*, she said; he actually thought that she wasn't attracted enough to him! Little did he know that, though she loved him, he was barely in Marie's thoughts at all when they slept together. Instead, her obsession with her weight remained front and center.

"Ironically," Marie told me with a harsh laugh, "the whole thing is eating me alive."

What makes you you? While you probably recognized aspects of your behavior in each of the five general descriptions in the previous chapter, the details of that behavior can belong only to one person. Where did Marie's come from? Where did *yours* come from?

In this chapter we'll be looking at the three sources that shape our stories about our sexual selves: nature, nurture, and culture. Along the way, we'll occasionally revisit Marie's story to see how these sources shaped her sexual self-image. I'd also like you to ask yourself how your sexual identity might have been shaped by your belief in individual stories about your own sexual life. You'll come to realize that your stories, although their details are particular to your experience, are not unlike Marie's stories about her sexual life, my stories about my sexual life, and everyone else's stories about their sexual lives.

THE THREE FACETS OF EVE

NATURE

From the moment a baby comes out of the womb and the doctor announces, "It's a girl!," there are certain wheels that are almost inevitably set in motion. The baby grows into a little girl who has ideas and fantasies about her vagina, based not only on looking at it, touching it, and comparing it with her mother's vagina but also on comparing it with its opposite: the penis.

Sigmund Freud started out saying that a girl is like a boy in every way until she realizes she doesn't have a penis, and from that moment on, her whole development revolves around the "missing" organ. Of course, Freud later went on to say that he hadn't studied children and that he actually didn't know what the hell he was talking about when it came to the childhood development of females. Still, in my experience, I do think most girls experience some combination of anxiety about their own genitals and envy of males' genitals.

Do you remember the Mister Rogers song about boys being "fancy on the outside" and girls being "fancy on the inside"? I suspect that even the well-intentioned, earnest, cardigan-wearing Mister Rogers was unable to completely reassure any little-girl viewer whose brother was whipping around the backyard with his penis out, aiming his stream of urine in a big arc, whooping it up and having a grand old time. In any case, I'm unable to completely reassure *my* 4-year-old daughter. . . .

At the moment, she's preoccupied with the idea of boys standing and peeing. She has wistfully told me how much better this is than her own situation, in which she has to sit down on a toilet to pee and can't see the place the pee is coming from, and it often dribbles down her leg instead of shooting out in one neat stream the way a boy's pee does. When my daughter complains to me that she can't do what a boy does, I tell her that I understand her feelings. I also tell her that she has a lot of parts down there, more parts than a boy. I say that when she touches her vagina it feels just as good as when a boy touches his penis, and I remind her time and again that boys and girls are different and that neither set of genitals is better than the other.

I tell myself that such a reasonable separate-but-equal explanation is probably not making much of a dent, for this simple reason: To a 4-year-old, bigger is better.

Suppose you give a 4-year-old two gift boxes: one very, very big, tied with a red ribbon, and one rather small and plain. Now suppose you say to her, "You can choose one box, but first let me tell you that the tiny one has something much cooler inside it!" Which one will she choose? Nine times out of 10, it'll be the big box.

In this case the big box isn't just bigger. It moves. She's no fool. She wants the thing that's big and moves and does tricks, yet she's left with this . . . this . . . indefinable space, this hole. This *nothing*, she might think.

Girls' experience of their genitals is opposed to that of boys, who unmistakably have a *something*. From a young age, they can't miss it. As soon as they're out of diapers, they have to learn to hold it in order to urinate. They can consider it from every angle—and they do. As far back as every man can remember, he's been on intimate terms with his penis, measuring it, touching it, probably even naming it. Every boy masturbates, unless he's told that his hands will fall off—and even then, he'll continue to masturbate (but just feel bad about it). Once he enters adolescence and sees how his penis responds to stimulation, even just idly thinking about blond-haired Sally Cannetti, who sits in the next row during algebra, it becomes an object of fascination, worthy of close study. If there were an SAT exam all about the penis, every man would ace it. (#3: Which way does your penis usually hang when it's inside your pants? #8: How long, when fully erect, would you say your penis is?)

For girls, however, a lot of what we've got is hidden from view, tucked away on the inside. Hey, what's in there, anyway? We can't see it, we can't peer inside, and therefore we are anxious about what we have. This aura of mystery and confusion extends to masturbation. If the vagina seems vague, then it won't be clear to us exactly where the sensations are coming from. We don't know where to touch or how to "flip the switch" in the place that would feel good. Many girls never put a hand there; instead they use a pillow or the corner of a counter. (Some of them grow up into women who have spent a lifetime without really knowing their vaginas, simply coexisting with them like two polite but distant roommates.)

To complicate matters further, at the age of 3 or 4 a girl will go through a period of individuation, of thinking, "I'm separate from Mommy; I'm my own person." A little boy at this age will go through his own period of figuring out that he's separate from his father, but as he does so he'll notice that though he may not look like Dad, the two of them do have the same apparatus. (Which doesn't mean that boys don't have their own insecurities and vulnerabilities about their penises, but the issues are different from what they are for girls.) For a little girl, such a connection with her mother is more difficult. She has no breasts like her mommy and there's no protruding genital organ to see; even the nonprotruding one that the mommy has, after all, is covered up in hair. When the little girl can't relate to her mother in this way, she might feel anxious, vulnerable, small, and unimportant.

You might say that I ought to tell my daughter that not only is her vagina special and different and fancy on the inside, but also it will one day be able to do an amazing thing that no penis has ever been able to do: give birth to a baby. That idea, however, is too abstract and absurd for a little girl to really take any comfort in. In fact, it's often frightening to dwell on this; how could a baby come out of that hole? Doesn't it hurt?

Even as girls get older, the sense of penis-versus-vagina doesn't get any easier. Once they become aware of penises—of their dad's penis, say—and begin to learn that the penis goes into the vagina, they become frightened. They think, quite reasonably, that it's got to hurt. After all, how can a tiny little vagina ever hold such a thing? That can't really work, can it?

So what's a mother (or a father) to do?

NURTURE

From the very start, the way your parents treat you and the way they respond to the whole subject of genitals is going to have a big impact.

Many parents never refer to the vagina or penis by name. They refer to the area "down there." Maybe the Place That Shall Not Be Named is not named because the mother herself isn't sure of her own anatomical structure. Maybe it's not named because the parents are simply uncomfortable with saying those names out loud. Either way, what kind of message does it send if this essential part of a child's life remains nameless? Imagine what you might grow up thinking if your parents referred to your entire intellectual life—your ability to learn in school and think about the future and begin to make decisions for yourself and take responsibility for your choice of words and deeds—as only "up there"!

Calling the genitals "down there" not only leaves them nameless but also smooshes together the whole kit and caboodle. When a parent opens a boy's diaper, there's usually a clear distinction between the urine in the front and the feces in the back, and therefore between penis and anus. Not so for a girl. Unless the parents clarify that the place where the pee comes out is different from the place where the smelly poop comes out, which in turn is different from the vulva and the clitoris and so on (most parents don't, because they're uncomfortable with naming parts), then the child might start to regard her genitals as one big mushy, stinky place.

Maybe you're thinking, "Well, okay . . . but the baby's still in diapers. How is anything that happens at that age going to affect her development?" An infant does have some vague and fuzzy awareness of her genitals. For instance, when you open the wet diaper and she feels the air on her skin, it feels good and gives her certain sensations. By age 2 she's taking notice of her genitals, essentially saying to herself: "Hey, this is mine! I'm a girl. I've got this whole package of stuff down here. I've got a vulva, and a clitoris, and a . . ." Well, okay, maybe no

2-year-old on earth ever said those things to herself. The point is, children routinely stay in diapers until at least their third birthday, definitely long enough for their parents' actions to register in their developing minds and make a difference.

Children's attitudes are formed by not only their parents' actions but also their own reactions. If Mom or Dad is disgusted by a dirty diaper, the baby girl might start to think that her genitals are somehow bad. It's hygienically important, of course, that people wash their hands after using the toilet, but parents who are overly anxious about this matter lead their kids to think "Wow, I must be really, really dirty down there."

Consider the damage this lesson can do later in life, when a young woman tries to claim her rightful place in the world of sexuality and these old memories kick in. How can she enjoy sex, an experience in which she'll need to reveal her vagina— that disgusting, dirty place—to another person?

Even if a parent is enlightened enough to call all the parts by their rightful names and to express no discomfort about what comes out of them, a negative attitude might still reveal itself to the impressionable child (and is there any other kind?). What are the parents' attitudes toward boys and girls, toward penises and vaginas?

First, let's look at the mother's possible responses. Pregnant women spend hours reading baby-name books, fantasizing about who that swelling belly is going to turn out to be. Often they have a strong fantasy about it being either a boy or a girl. They are positive they know which sex the baby is, even without an ultrasound or amnio. These strong fantasies are either

realized or dashed the moment the baby is delivered. Sometimes, the effects of having a baby of the "wrong" sex can rever-
berate as that baby grows up.

For instance, a mother might have privately hoped for a
boy. Maybe boys were more highly valued in her family, as is
the case in some cultures. This mother might never have come
right out and told her daughter of her disappointment, but
there are subtle ways in which the daughter might pick up the
truth. A mother doesn't have to dress her little girl in blue all
the time in order for the daughter to sense that who she is, and
what she possesses, may not be good enough. Parents express
their real feelings in all kinds of unconscious ways. Even when
we think we're keeping feelings inside, somehow they slip out
without our knowing it.

If a mother is uncomfortable or unhappy with her own sexuality (and so, for example, doesn't dignify body parts by calling them by their proper names), then she'll automatically
convey that in some way to her daughter. The daughter will
pick up the unconscious coded message and apply it to her own
body and her feelings about herself as a female. The way the
mother and father relate to each other, which has nothing to do
with their child at all, also passes on a clear message to their
daughter that she applies directly to her own sexual self.

You see how the trap is set, then sprung again and again,
generation after generation: The little girl gets older, harboring
her own (often wrongheaded) feelings about her genitals, how
they operate, how aesthetically pleasing they are (or aren't),
whether they're as good as a boy's, and so on. It isn't until

puberty that her mother usually tries to clarify some of the most pressing issues. So one day in marches Mom with a humiliating jumbo pink box of Stayfree Maxi pads, and she's beaming and telling her daughter, "Congratulations, you're a woman now," and trying to share with her daughter her own feelings that she remembers from the first time she herself menstruated. When I was growing up, for instance, our gym teacher sent the boys off to play dodgeball, then showed the girls in our class a short film about a girl named Naomi who wants a yellow dress she sees in the window of a store. Her mother says she's not ready for it because the dress is kind of revealing and adult. By the end of this (creaky but sweet) little film, we've seen a diagram of the female reproductive system and learned about all the "wonderful" things that are happening inside a pubescent girl's body. In the last scene of the film—surprise, surprise—Naomi is allowed to buy that dress!

In real life, the big talk that the mother initiates with her daughter is more often than not met with a kind of frozen, silent horror. Gone is the little girl whose body didn't resemble her mother's at all, and in its place is a body that, minus a bit of cellulite perhaps, finally does resemble her mother's. Along with the daughter's development come new negative feelings, such as "Will my mom be mad at me?" and "Do I have permission to be sexual?" The two women are suddenly, in a way, rivals for the attentions of men. They are now competing in the same universe.

The mother may wax poetic about menstruation, but her daughter can't get out of the room fast enough. This attitude is an echo of what her mother did to her a long time ago, when the little girl needed reassurance about her own inadequacies about her genitals, and the mother was embarrassed and hemmed and hawed and couldn't get out of that room fast enough. The daughter has by now internalized the mother's message, which is essentially that there's something wrong with talking about the whole "down there" issue, and that there's something wrong with "down there" altogether.

Now, needing information, where does this newly pubescent girl go? Why, to her friends at school, of course, which is essentially a case of the blind leading the blind. You may remember from your own puberty that it's usually the so-called "bad girls" who possess the most information about sex. The girls who are being overly sexual or taking lots of risks with their bodies are often the sources of information. Therefore, the girl who needs information but was unable to listen to her mom thinks to herself, "It's the dirty girls who know the most." This reinforces the whole notion that anything having to do with the vagina is just plain bad.

It's an endless cycle, a hamster wheel of shame and guilt and general discomfort. For many women, the wheel will turn and turn for many, many years.

Where is the dad in all this? A father is often no less invested in the sex of the baby than the mother is and can show his delight or disappointment in the same subtle, unconscious ways. He can unwittingly contribute to a daughter's sense of inadequacy by chuckling and making a fuss about a son's ability to "point and shoot," which he remembers fondly from his own childhood. Since there's no parallel praise and fuss for anything a little girl can do with her vagina, she's left to feel embarrassed or simply ordinary.

The ways in which parents pass along their attitudes about the differences between the sexes extend beyond discussions about penises and vaginas. These beliefs wrap themselves in various hiding-in-plain-sight disguises throughout daily life. In Marie's case, her mother clearly thought that separate rules applied to women and men. Women had to be hypervigilant about their appearances, imprisoning themselves (like "jail-birds") in worries about weight and other aspects of body image, while men got to wander outside the prison grounds, roaming the free world, buttering their bread, and doing whatever else they pleased to—and with—their bodies. This us-and-them approach was only reinforced by Marie's father, who gladly indulged himself and established himself as the role model for his son.

What childhood experiences of yours might have taken psychic tolls? How did your parents treat sex, either the body parts or body image? What about your siblings? What early influences might still be affecting your vision of yourself in ways that you've never thought about, never really realized (until you picked up this book, that is)?

CULTURE

We live not only inside our bodies and inside the houses in which we were raised but also in the world. Our culture creates the third powerful influence on a young girl's view of her sexual self. Society's view of sex is inescapable. It is everywhere and it often contains shockingly damaging ideas.

When I was a young doctor starting out in my psychiatric residency, I was rigorously immersed in all kinds of subjects. I was trained in pathology, medications, and other crucial topics. There was one subject, however, that went almost without mention. It amazed me how rarely any of the people training us brought up sexuality. Of course, when we became practicing psychiatrists ourselves, we would need to be able to feel comfortable talking with our patients about their sex lives, but the people training us weren't comfortable. What kind of message did that send?

Everywhere you go in life, you find yourself confronting other people's discomfort with sexuality. It's all over the place: among parents and teachers and kids. From looking at American TV shows and movies, you'd think we live in a freewheeling culture that accepts sex. Not so. The volume of sexual and sensationalistic material that's out there bears no relation to the attitudes we carry within our deepest selves. I've encountered it myself while preparing for an appearance on a network television news show: "You can't say the word 'orgasm' on TV at 7:30 in the morning!" It's as if adults can't be reminded first thing in the morning of what they did last thing last night. We might watch porn on the Internet, but we still feel our sexual organs are dirty and embarrassing. We might tell off-color jokes largely to deflect our own great uneasiness about the subjects these jokes address.

I felt it was a necessary part of my professional training to try to resolve this disconnect, so one year I did a fellowship in sexual dysfunction. Here I dealt with the real problems that men and women encounter in the bedroom. There were men who couldn't get erections and women for whom intercourse was painful. A very small subset of the residents took part in this fellowship, and it gave me the first chance I'd ever had as a doctor to ask certain questions. We spent hours talking about vaginas and clitorises, looking into the medical causes of sexual dysfunction. The words flew fast and loose around the room.

I admit that when I embarked upon my fellowship, I felt interested but uncomfortable. I'd grown up in a household that was pretty progressive, at least compared to those of my friends. Even so, sitting with a group of men and women in white coats, the topic seemed novel, unusual, a little illicit, especially when we moved away from medical aspects and started talking about emotional and psychological components. Generally, doctors are more comfortable looking at something in a clinical way. We would rather say "What about the spasms in the outer third of your vagina?" than "Let's talk about how you feel about your vagina."

Doctors are uncomfortable, and women are uncomfortable, too. As a doctor, I wish I could simply prescribe a cure for society's uptight and shamefaced nature. Correcting or reversing these ideas would be a formidable task, because so many of the bad messages start and are embedded early. When girls embark on their lives as teenagers, complete with menstrual cramps and acne and crushes and desires, they bring with them a lot of baggage, including Samsonite's full Inadequacy line. At this extremely vulnerable time, these teens are bombarded with messages in the media about what it takes to be a sexy woman and attract men. Being considered sexy, in the mass media, isn't usually about being powerful but about looking like a phallic equivalent. (Don't roll your eyes. Just take a look at some of those women in *Vogue* or those celebrities in *People*, and check out their impossibly long silhouettes and their stiletto heels.) We want our models and stars to be tall as trees, to grow upward. We want them to look like flashy, expensively dressed, Manolo Blahnik–wearing penises.

Is it any wonder that women today learn to believe that image is everything and that feeling powerful inside isn't important? Rather than trying to feel cool and sexy and strong within, young women wonder how they appear to others and they try to do what they can to control and regulate that—and *only* that—set of appearances.

Recent studies have shown just how extreme the negative ripple effects from popular culture can be. Girls who identify with the increasingly exploitive images of women in movies, magazines, cable TV, and the Internet don't think of sexuality as related to intimacy. Instead, they wind up seeing themselves as society sees those women: as objects. Ironically, these girls' efforts to make themselves cool and desirable only leave them with lower self-esteem and higher rates of depression and eating disorders.

Unfortunately, this sorry situation only gets worse as time passes. Past 18, young women's bodies will start to show some of the effects of gravity. When women are in their early twenties, things really begin to change. Matters are further complicated by childbirth, when and if it occurs. At that point, many women, taught that their value rests in their perfect bodies, feel as though they might as well curl up in a ball or wear a thick sweater and a hat pulled over their faces for the rest of their lives.

The cycle doesn't end when women enter their thirties, forties, fifties, and beyond. Young women who internalize society's ideas about the perfect body become older women who look at their aging bodies not with appreciation of their own strength and physical capabilities but with disgust and sadness at the toll that time, childbearing, menopause, and other ups and downs take on their previously full breasts and firm thighs.

It may surprise you to learn that men are often more comfortable talking about the vagina than women are. Men love your vagina! They love it far more than you do. They appreciate its taste and its smell, they aren't ashamed of it, and they like to think about it during the day and remember the sensations it brings out in them.

What's more, many men happen to be sexually turned on by a pendulous breast or a curvy hip. Believe it or not, plenty of men are not looking for some emaciated 18-year-old waif and would in fact vastly prefer someone else entirely. Society idealizes the stick-thin model, but men often love the soft and sensual dimensions of the grown female body. Philip truly appreciated Marie, but she didn't know what to do with him. She couldn't even imagine that such a man could exist. By day she flipped through fashion magazines; by night she cowered under the covers.

The impact of culture on our ideas about sexuality extends beyond physical appearances. Assumptions about which sex is stronger, and even about what strength means, are part of every society that humans have ever managed to create. Is the person who raises a child who can make a positive contribution to society stronger than the person who makes a killing in the stock market? It's easy to say that ideally both images of strength have merit, but the reality is that at any point in history we do tend to value one kind of image over the other, even if those values shift over time.

In recent years, we have seen these values shifting almost right before our eyes. More women have begun working outside the home than ever before and more women have achieved high-power jobs than ever before. As a result, women are sometimes able to make more money or achieve higher status than their husbands. For some couples, such a shift is difficult. Even couples who see themselves as enlightened or evolved might unconsciously still struggle with a situation where the man is more the keeper of the home and kids while the woman has the greater presence (and earning potential) in the world.

It's easy to imagine how a man in this situation might feel some diminishment of his masculinity. Even the woman who tries not to see him this way—who can afford to be emotionally generous and sympathetic—might not be able to overcome a lifetime of traditional masculine/feminine role-playing. The more she sees herself as powerful, aggressive, and strong, the more she might not see him in those terms, at least compared to herself. Maybe in her unconscious fantasy world what remains sexy is a strong powerful man who "takes her," who overpowers her; a man whom she can depend on, turn to, and be enveloped in. (Think of Harlequin romances; there's a reason their popularity endures.) The more she sees her mate as less masculine and herself as more masculine, the less sexually exciting being with him in bed might seem.

This situation is not as uncommon as you or I might wish. Many women take out their frustration and anger by belittling their partners further. "Can't you even fix the roof while I am out supporting this family?" "Can't you even pick up the house while I have that important meeting?" I'm not saying that the housekeeping should revert to an earlier generation's unfair division of labor, with the "head of the household" not lifting a finger. A feeling of fairness is crucial in a marriage and needs to be maintained. A woman who wants a macho guy in bed will have to help him be one without patronizing him or compromising her own feelings of achievement. If that means helping him to fill a masculine role that's more traditional than the relationship, then my advice is: Do it!

The woman in such a partnership can start during the day, rather than waiting for bed. She can tell him that he's sexy when he takes off his shirt and chops that wood—because he is! She might go for a drive with him at the wheel with his arm around her. The point is to allow and create scenarios that are consistent with a sexual fantasy life—and with sexual tension—that the couple can later summon up in the bedroom.

Wʜᴇɴ ᴄᴏɴsɪᴅᴇʀɪɴɢ ᴛʜᴇ ɪɴꜰʟᴜᴇɴᴄᴇs ᴏꜰ nature, nurture, or culture on your sexual identity, the bottom line is that you can't predict what someone else will like, so you may as well be someone *you* like and take care of the body you have. Nobody would suggest that Marie should "let herself go," but she did find Philip, who appreciated her for what she was and how she looked. Marie couldn't appreciate herself, and it was her response to that self-image that crept into bed with her and Philip at night, ruining the moment and threatening the relationship—at least until Marie began to understand the influences that had shaped her negative self-image, the stories that seemed to be "eating her alive."

Personal and cultural histories combine to influence how you see yourself sexually—accurately or, far too often, not. Now the time has come for you to follow Marie's example and figure out exactly who that imaginary someone is—and how to change her story.

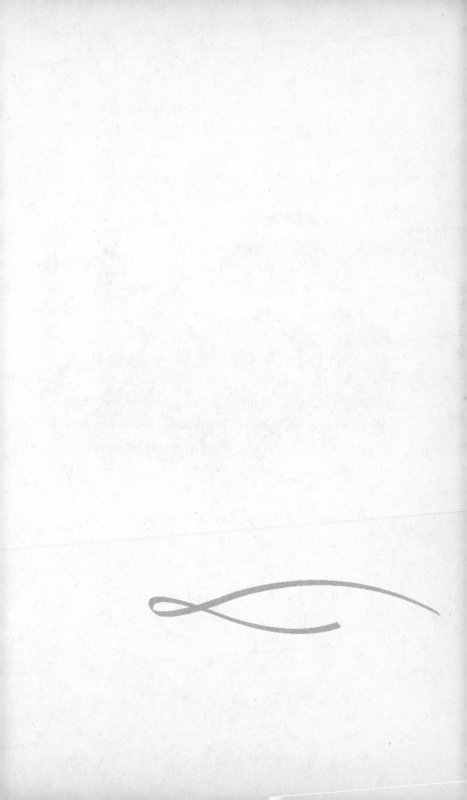

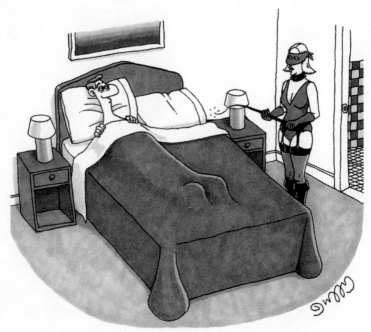

"Please listen carefully, as my menu options have changed."

CHAPTER THREE

CREATING YOUR OWN RIPPLE EFFECT

ADDY WAS A PATIENT WHO WAS LIKE many women I know: in her early forties, warm, overworked, crazy about her kids. For several weeks my conversations with her were general and vague, despite my attempts to get her to be specific about various aspects of her life. One day I could see that she was clearly upset as soon as she sat down. She wanted to talk. No, she *needed* to talk.

"Something happened," Maddy said right away and she didn't need any encouragement to keep going. "Our anniversary was last weekend, and it was my idea we go somewhere."

What she described sounded like an idyllic romantic getaway: a weekend at an inn in Connecticut, no kids, no cell phones, no work, just her and her husband, Mark. Friday started with a great dinner, then Maddy and Mark went for a walk, watched the sunset, and went to bed. They were lying in a giant four-poster, starting to "fool around," as Maddy said, when out of the corner of her eye she noticed that Mark hadn't folded his shirt and pants but had left them bunched up on the rocking chair across the room.

This got to her.

She tried making light of it. "Come on, big boy," she said, "why don't you go over there and fold your clothes first?" Mark wasn't amused. He sat up in bed and said that she ruined any moment of intimacy they ever had anymore. He told her that basically she was sabotaging their sex life.

When she reached this point in her story, Maddy feigned amusement for a moment, as if the very idea that any woman might sabotage her sex life was absurd, and then her face crumpled. She burst into tears, then looked up at me, her eyes blazing. "I told him that was ridiculous. But you know what? I think he's right." She pulled a tissue from the box on the table in front of her. "We made up later that night," she went on softly. "Everything's fine again, and neither of us has mentioned it again. But what I did—and what he said about it—I just can't stop thinking about it."

HOW WE GET OUR STORIES

At some point during the weeks or months of therapy sessions in my office, a patient will find herself confronting an uncomfortable truth. She'll squirm a little, and then she'll inevitably ask a version of this question: "Who, me?"

"Yes, you," I always want to say. "Yes, us—all of us."

Which means, yes, you, too.

Whatever your individual issues may be, they are familiar to me. They would be familiar to any competent therapist. We therapists like to say to one another that we've heard it all, and, in fact, those of us who have been around long enough pretty much have. Not only that, we *want* to hear it all. We want to hear every facet of the problems a patient is facing, and we want to hear the problems described as accurately and, if need be, as forcefully as possible. Even if a patient wants to shout at us and tell us to go to hell, we want to hear it. Honest. Such a response just might be an indication that we're getting close to something significant.

I want to be clear here. To say that what you think about your sexuality fits one or more of five common patterns or to say that they would be familiar to any competent therapist doesn't diminish them in the least. These types don't mean you're the same as everyone else in that category. They don't make you like anyone else and they don't make you any less *you*. All they mean is that you share certain traits and certain common struggles with other women. At any moment in your life, the particular combination of this-much-from-this-category and that-much-from-that-category and a-pinch-of-this-other-category is a combination that belongs to no one else. It's the unique recipe for you.

It's not just the combination of details that defines you. It's the individual details themselves. Perhaps you've heard the expression that the devil is in the details. Maybe you've also heard the expression that God is in the details. Both apply here. Only by confronting your demons (so to speak) will you find salvation (so to speak).

Getting at those details can be difficult. Shame and embarrassment are powerful obstacles to emotional health. It's one thing for you to hear me say that our individual stories about our sexual selves arise through numberless influences in our culture and personal experiences. It's quite another for you to say, "These are *my* stories"—to know where they came from and what they mean.

Consider Maddy and her response to her husband's unfolded clothes. Her story touched me, but it didn't surprise me. It was clear to me right away, as it was to her husband, that Maddy's sabotage of her romantic weekend wasn't just an isolated incident. It was chronic, and it was serving some kind of purpose, even if she had no idea what that purpose was. She had her reasons, reasons she and I eventually uncovered, but they don't concern us yet. What concerns us instead is how *you* would respond to the sight of your partner's shirt and pants and underwear and socks tossed casually over a chair. How would you respond if you happened to see it right in the middle of lovemaking? Would you offer criticism and risk ruining the moment? Would you care about the clothes at all? Would you even notice?

Maddy noticed, cared, and criticized. And that's Maddy. That's who she is. The fact that she had those responses, out of all the variety and combination of responses in the world, is what makes her *her*.

The responses that you would have had in that same situation are what makes you *you*. All day, every day, you're responding. Ten excess pounds? No problem. Just more of you to love. Ten excess pounds? Big problem. Nobody could ever love a body like that. Oily T-zone? Simple: You apply some astringent and some makeup, put on your best smile, and go out to dinner. Or: You cancel the evening, pile on the facial mud mask, and crawl under the covers. Your partner nearing orgasm: a source of pulse-quickening excitement in yourself and a soul-exchanging unity with your partner, or a good opportunity to ponder whether tomorrow night's grilled salmon would go well with a bottle of Pinot Grigio?

What's at stake isn't who takes out the garbage, gets up with the kids, makes dinner, or does the grocery shopping. It's not the love handles, the oily T-zone, the hot flashes, or the sagging breasts. It's not your vagina.

More accurately, it's all those things. In everyday life they are indeed the details we need to deal with, but what's at stake isn't *only* all those things. They make up only the surface of a life. What's happening under the surface? What do these seemingly ordinary, everyday things mean? What do they mean to *you?* Yes, the argument is about the garbage or the groceries, but, more important, it's about where your specific responses come from. It's about a specific source, a part of you that harbors all the thoughts and feelings outside your awareness. It's about your unconscious.

It would be an overstatement to say that the unconscious is absolutely everything we're not aware of. We are, each of us, part nature as expressed by an individual genetic code and brain chemistry. I might be more sensitive to the sound of fingernails on a blackboard than you are, and you might have a faster metabolism than I do. One girl might reach puberty at 12, another at 15. A woman might hit menopause at 45 or 50 or 55. Yet in addition to these natural differences, we are all subject to our common instincts. When we're hungry, we eat. When we're tired, we sleep. When we see a person we find sexy, we go hubba-hubba and we go more hubba-hubba or less hubba-hubba according to our hormone levels.

We're also part nurture, shaped by the behaviors and belief systems we've internalized from constant exposure to our families, our friends, and society at large. As Maddy and I talked over the course of weeks, we came to understand that for her, sex was accompanied by a constant refrain: her mother's voice. Maddy's mother had actually died 12 years before Maddy came to see me, but that didn't matter. There the voice was, in Maddy's head, just as it had been when she was a 6-year-old girl lying in bed in her comfortable suburban home. Back then, the voice was saying that if you touched yourself, you were bad. Back then, what Maddy would do is lie in the dark and try not to touch herself, because she didn't want to be bad, yet there was her hand, moving as if by its own will, drifting along the outside of her pajamas, touching the top of her thigh, and "accidentally" brushing up against her groin. Then it accidentally brushed her groin again and again.

Maddy would wrest her hand away and lie still, arms straight, hands at her sides. "Who would want to touch that hole, anyway? Who touches holes? It's just a stupid hole where the pee comes out and where, later on, babies somehow come out, too," though that made no sense to her. How could they possibly fit? Maddy would continue to lie there, both hands unmoving, heavy as anvils.

When Maddy told me this story, it all began to make sense. How now she didn't think about anything during sex. How she waited for her husband to be done and for sex to be over. How, as far as she was concerned, her vagina was still nothing more than a hole. How her sexual identity was also just one big, general "down there."

This memory of lying awake in her childhood bedroom wasn't just *a* story. It was *her* story. "I'm bad": This was the lesson of the story that Maddy would carry within her throughout her life and that would define her sexuality to this day. To a large extent, Maddy still was that 6-year-old lying awake in her suburban bedroom, at least as far as her sense of her sexual self was concerned. No wonder she responded the way she did to her own sexuality, to say nothing of her husband's advances! In Maddy's world, her husband's sexual desires were an imposition, a lack of consideration, an obliviousness to her very presence—not unlike a pile of unfolded clothes.

I'm not suggesting that Maddy actually heard her mother's voice. She wasn't delusional. Maddy wasn't even aware that the voice of her mother had become such a dominant feature of her life. It took the two of us a long time and a lot of work to get to the point where Maddy could even recall this memory, let alone admit to herself that it had caused so many problems throughout her life, continuing to this day. Without realizing it, Maddy, like so many women, had segregated her sexual side from the rest of herself. In rejecting her husband's sexual advances, she was basically rejecting her own sexuality. She was turning away from the crucial part of her that contained the possibility of pleasure, grace, power, and well-being.

How could something that she could barely even remember have such an effect on her? That's where the unconscious comes in. The unconscious isn't just a repository for the thoughts and impulses that lie outside our consciousness. The unconscious doesn't just sit there, doing nothing. Despite its seeming absence, it is an active *presence*. It's doing something all the time: It is surrounding you with the stories of your life.

In order to make sense of the way we see the world now, we have no choice but to draw on earlier interpretations of similar experiences. After all, they're all we've got! We see the world now in the ways we saw the world then, at that time in our lives. We draw on those interpretations because they made sense then and they continue to make sense now. They exert a hold on us because they seem to us like the real world.

We all see pretty much the same world: the same oily T-zone, the same pile of unfolded clothes. What those images mean to each of us, the significance that we find in what we see, is unique. Your world is not the same as my world, and my world isn't the same as Maddy's, and on and on. We each respond to every set of circumstances according to an individual interpretation. Those interpretations will continue to seem like the real world unless we can recognize that they're not—that they are, instead, simply the stories that make up our lives.

Now, not all these stories create problems. Your stories might make you ambitious, generous, sympathetic, or loving. When your stories affect you in ways that hurt you and make you want to change, as they certainly did in Maddy's case, then the time has come to realize that they're not a reflection of the way the world has to be. The time has come to recognize them and to overcome them—to change the ripple effect emanating from your sexuality from a negative influence to a positive influence.

How will you know that the time has come?

WHY WE CHANGE OUR STORIES

What makes you *you* is that out of all the combinations of emotional responses in the world, you respond to a situation with one individual set of responses. If that set of responses comes from all the vast and various influences that you've experienced throughout your life, then the next logical question is: Why now? Why are those responses creating trouble for your personal life *now?*

In this section we're going to be asking three basic questions. Why has this combination of responses surfaced right now? Why has this combination of responses surfaced with such urgency right now? Why have you decided to deal with your emotional responses right now?

The answer in each case is the same: Something happened.

What something? "You tell me," I say to my patients. On the page, of course, you and I don't have the luxury of a personal dialogue, so I'll say this to you, instead: "You tell yourself."

To help you consider that challenge, try thinking of this "something that happened" in terms of an idea I often use in my practice: trigger point. I like this term because it brings to mind a provocative image—a finger slowly squeezing the trigger of a gun, the physical pressure building up much like the emotional pressure inside you. Sometimes the finger loosens its grip, the emotions recede, and the gun doesn't go off, but sometimes you trip the trigger, and all hell breaks loose.

In trying to figure out why, you can ask yourself these three questions:

Why has this combination of responses surfaced right now?

This is probably the easiest of the three questions to answer, though you're the only one who can answer it. Can you think of an instance when a set of challenging and perhaps conflicting emotions suddenly rose to the surface? Whatever it is should be knowable to you, perhaps even painfully obvious. The issues might be traits you don't like, patterns that defeat you, an aspect of your own personality you wouldn't want to encounter in a stranger, and problems that just won't go away. What all of these issues have in common is that they're recurring. They've happened again and again in your life, and now they're happening one more time. In trying to identify the trigger point that has brought these sets of emotional responses to the surface at one particular moment, your job is to ask yourself: Where have I seen this before?

**Why has this combination of responses surfaced with
such urgency right now?**

Once you feel you've figured out where you've seen this particular issue before, what circumstances might have triggered it
on those various occasions, and, therefore, what similar circumstances may have triggered it now, you need to ask yourself why
it's surfaced so forcefully that you feel you must fix it.

Sometimes the answer is obvious. A major life change for a
woman can bring any number of emotions to the surface. For
some women, pregnancy serves as a reminder of lost youth. For
others, it represents a fulfillment of purpose. For some women,
it's a cause of anxiety about leaving behind the cultural norm
of slinky sexiness. For others, it's a way of becoming as powerful as their mothers, a dynamic that itself can cut both ways.
Consider menopause. Of course, it often carries a message of
lost fertility. If the woman's mother had trouble growing old
gracefully, then chances are the daughter will face the same
problem when her time comes. When entering menopause, one
woman might feel: Who would want this shriveled, dry old
body? Another woman entering menopause might look forward
to freedom from birth control, a liberation that itself might
accompany that time of life when the children leave the house
and a couple has the place to themselves for the first time in a
couple of decades. Suddenly they're not worrying about the
kids barging in or overhearing troublesome noises and they can
take their time. Suddenly time is on their side.

Of course, a woman might experience conflicting emotions:
not only happiness at being pregnant but also sorrow at the loss
of a youthful figure; wistfulness at reaching menopause and

watching her children leave home but satisfaction at returning to an earlier sense of freedom.

Not every life change need be major. Maddy went ballistic when her husband tossed his clothes onto a chair during a weekend getaway. The sight of her husband's sloppiness was her trigger point. That kind of extreme response might sound petty at first, but it's actually not. For Maddy, her husband's sloppiness was a pretext for her to keep on doing what she'd been doing all along—avoiding intimacy. In this moment, though, it erupted because she was experiencing a perfect storm of emotions. Because she and her husband had deliberately planned a weekend of nothing but intimacy, Maddy found she had nowhere to run. She had none of the little excuses she might have used on a daily (or nightly) basis. This was it: naked intimacy, front and center. For you or me, or even for Maddy on another day in another place, a pile of clothes might have been just a pile of clothes, but on this day in this bed, that bunch of innocent fabric became a major trigger point in her life.

Even a major trigger point in itself isn't always enough to force you to confront a recurring problem.

Why have you decided to deal with your emotional responses right now?

Logically speaking, when a trigger point has created some sort of crisis in your life, you should try to figure out why you're continuing to behave in a certain way. Being logical has nothing to do with your actual response. When you're dealing with the unconscious, you're actually dealing with an absence of reason.

Here you are, trying to figure out why you continue to behave in certain ways. Wouldn't it be easier not to try to find out? Why bother wrestling with such difficult, daunting issues? Why be willing to subject yourself to the discomfort of discovering a potentially difficult truth about yourself? Why be willing to confront failings, admit mistakes, strip away illusions that so far have made your life bearable?

For the same reason that so many women make their way to my office and many women who are already my patients find themselves finally admitting to themselves and to me that they need help in ways they'd previously denied. In some way, a life lived according to untruths and evasions, however comforting they've been in the past, has become unbearable, or at least less bearable than a life lived *not* according to untruths and evasions, a life lived honestly and truthfully.

The trigger point might have been obvious or even might have been predictable—pregnancy, menopause. Sometimes, though, seemingly minor trigger points can assume major importance precisely because, at first, they seem easier to deal with. They seem important but almost beside the point, so the patient doesn't feel threatened and feels free to put all her emotional energy into it. Only then does the major issue surface. Maddy thought she needed to talk about intimacy—not her mother's hectoring voice.

What about you? Has anything happened in your life to tip the balance between a life lived according to an untrue story that you've always blindly followed and a life lived by being honest with yourself? Something that perhaps prompted you to pick up this very book? I suspect so, and I wouldn't be surprised if you now suspect so, too. Something must have changed your attitude toward your sexual self to such an extent that you now want to know the truth about it, rather than continuing to rely on the stories you've always told yourself. Somewhere along the way you reached a trigger point so fundamentally important that it led you to want to change the most powerful sexual organ of all, your mind.

That brings us to the end of the three questions I would be asking you if you walked into my office. Now I'll give you a freebie. Here's a question you might wish you could ask me:

Why do I need to know what my trigger point is?

Shouldn't it be enough just to know that you want to change and that something has happened to make you want to change? The answer is a resounding no. It's not enough just to know that something has tripped your trigger. It's important to know why, and the trigger point can provide a clue. It's raw data. It's the DNA a CSI team wouldn't dream of throwing away. It's *your* DNA, psychologically speaking. What tripped your trigger wouldn't trip my trigger or Maddy's. It tripped your trigger because it's *your* trigger.

Knowing what the trigger is can be a significant first step toward knowing what it means to you, and knowing what it means to you can be the key to uncovering and understanding the stories that have shaped you. You'll need that key in order to take the pivotal step of changing how you see your sexuality.

HOW WE'LL CHANGE YOUR STORIES

Before we begin looking at the five types of stories in detail, I just want to give you a gentle reminder. A pep talk, really.

It's incredibly difficult, this whole taking-control-of-your-life process. It requires a lot of effort and concentration and perseverance. It requires a lot of commitment. In a way, it's a full-time job, and maybe you already have a full-time job. At some point, you're going to ask yourself whether it's actually worth all the trouble. That's a natural question. Everyone asks it. These beliefs from our past are very strong; they have to be, or else they wouldn't rule our lives the way they do.

Think of it this way: Just as you might try to change yourself physically by starting a diet or taking up cardio-boxing, so you can try to change yourself psychologically by finding healthier ways to think. Is sticking to a diet difficult? What about going to the gym four times a week? Of course! If you stay with the program, the result is that you feel better about your outward appearance and your whole life. The same is true here. If you stick with the program in this book, you'll feel better about your inward appearance and your whole life, though in a far more meaningful and lasting way than losing a few pounds or getting buff.

As incentive to get you started, I want to tell you that you're already further along than you might imagine. Don't you sometimes know what some friend's response is going to be, even before she opens her mouth? Can't you pretty much predict certain reactions from your parents, your partner, or your children? From yourself?

Of course you do. Of course you can. Consider this comment: "Look, as a friend, I just want to say that I know how hard you've been trying to lose those 10 pounds you put on after Anjelica was born. Don't hate me for saying this, and maybe it's none of my business anyway, but do you really think we should be ordering dessert?" You know the drill: A comment you could make to one friend, figuring that she'd see it as supportive, is a comment you wouldn't dare say to another friend, because you know she'd see it as criticism.

The same is true of you. You know how you would respond to most comments, most situations, don't you? You no doubt find yourself attracted to a certain type of person. You respond to a certain kind of physical appearance, combined with a certain mix of personality traits. At various points in your life you've probably found yourself responding to a possible mate. It's what you do without even thinking.

In the chapters to come, I'm going to ask you to do it *while* thinking. This is what I ask my patients to do. You and I won't be in the same room, of course, but at least we'll be on the same page. Together we'll discover what you already know about yourself without realizing you know it. In that way you will begin to ask yourself: What are my stories?

You'll very likely recognize yourself in the stories in each of the next five chapters. The five stories are representative of the most common stories that women tell themselves at one time or another in their sexual lives. In identifying, examining, and changing those stories, we'll follow a simple, direct format. I hope that by clearly laying out the information about who these women are, I can help you identify which stories influence your view of your sexual identity. After I tell you the story of a representative woman, as I did with Maddy, I'll take you step-by-step through how that representative woman got to be the sexual adult she is today and what she can do about that. All the while, I'll be encouraging you to consider how *you* got to be the sexual adult you are today and what *you* can do about that.

I'll start with How She Got That Story. We'll look at the *symptoms* this particular woman often exhibits, the patterns that make her her. Next, I'll cover the *sources* of those symptoms. Because all women are born with the same sexual goods, I won't dwell much on nature. Rather, I'll take the observations about nature that I made in Chapter 2 and show how they are reinforced by *nurture* and *culture* to create a particular category of symptoms.

I'll cover Why She Changed That Story. I'll discuss what might lead that woman to begin to recognize her problem and maybe even to seek help—what I call the *trigger point*. After all, her story has not only found an unproductive home in her *sex life* but also has radiated outward in a *ripple effect* that has affected her entire life.

We'll look at How to Change Your Story. We'll discuss the strategies that will let you take control of your sex life.

Finally, we'll see how by changing the story that controls your sex life, you will be Creating Your Own Ripple Effect—one that will radiate outward throughout your life and help transform you from the woman you are to the woman you want to be.

Who, you? Yes, you.

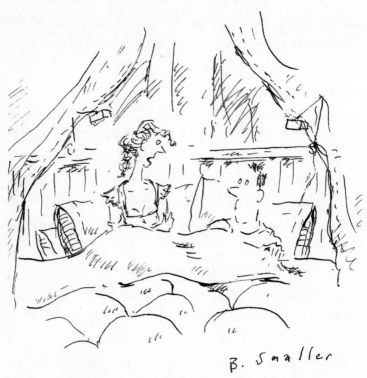

"Couldn't you at least try and read my mind?"

CHAPTER FOUR

WHEN YOU THINK YOU DON'T KNOW WHAT YOU'RE DOING

JENNY WAS 32 YEARS OLD, AND SHE HAD never once stood before a mirror and thought, "I like what I see." Her friends considered her a good-looking woman with cheekbones to die for and great legs, but Jenny couldn't share that view. She felt that something was intrinsically wrong with her and that everyone else knew it, too, but that they were just being kind to her. Jenny lived in a kind of bubble of self-delusion, and it affected almost every aspect of her daily life, including her work life, her emotional life, and, as she and I came to learn, her sexual life. When she first came to see me, she could speak only in the vaguest terms about a feeling of dissatisfaction.

This was a situation I found immediately familiar. Sometimes women are embarrassed to get too specific about what's bothering them. Other times, they actually don't know why they feel so bad. Either way, the sensation they describe is amorphous, a cartoon cloud that hangs over them and follows them around all day from their homes to their offices to their beds. For Jenny, as she wound up telling me during our initial session, after struggling to find just the right word, the cloud shadowing her every step took the form of embarrassment.

No matter how well she maintained her weight or how professionally she applied her makeup, she always had the uneasy sense that something wasn't right—that she was in some way ungainly or unsightly and everyone knew it, but no one would dare tell her. She'd never before said these thoughts aloud, she told me; she said she supposed they were just *there,* and always had been there, and she also said she supposed that that's why she was *here.* "And, you know," she added, "they're true."

She said this last word as if all I had to do to be convinced was to look at her. I looked. I saw a woman who wasn't overweight. I saw a woman who wasn't unattractive. I suspected I saw a woman who was far more critical of herself than she would ever be of her friends. She was the kind of woman who, when she was done getting dressed and putting on makeup, would stand before the mirror for one last look and sigh, as if to say that there was nothing more that could be done and, oh well, it was time to go to work.

Jenny was an adjunct faculty member in the communications department at a small college and even though part of her responsibility was to contribute to the conversation during faculty meetings, she found it difficult to do so. She felt she had nothing to add at these meetings. She felt her colleagues were far more articulate than she was and that if they found out how little she really knew, she'd be cast out into the street. I left the conversation there, not wanting to push her on our first meeting. A few sessions later Jenny was ready to tell me the way her feelings of inadequacy and even abnormality followed her into the bedroom, whenever she found herself sexually engaging with her boyfriend. "I just can't relax in bed," she confided. "I see these movies where women are totally comfortable while they have sex, like they were born knowing how to do it. Even after the sex is over, they lie there with their lovers and joke around, completely naked, their breasts and pubic hair and body fat and everything showing, not feeling at all self-conscious about how they look."

"Maybe not their body fat," I said. "Or pubic hair. That's not quite the Hollywood style."

Jenny gave a soft laugh. "Okay, maybe that says more about me than what's actually in the movies, but it is how I feel," she said. For Jenny, sex with her live-in boyfriend, Ed, was the same as it had been with all the other men she'd slept with: nothing like the way she'd heard it should be. She wasn't even sure if she experienced orgasms. She could get aroused, but she never really understood how to *know* if she'd had an orgasm—though she did know how to fake one, just as she knew how to fake her way through faculty meetings.

For Jenny, the physical facts of her sexuality were a mystery—a mystery she wasn't eager to explore. She knew that sexual sensations and orgasms are supposed to come from the clitoris. She didn't know if hers was normal—if it worked the way it was supposed to. She assumed it didn't, and she'd given it an apt nickname: "my nonworking doorbell."

Compared to women, Jenny figured, men have it easy. It's as if they're born knowing how to operate their equipment. Why not? Their sexual organs are right in the open, easy to reach, easy to examine, easy to get to know on an intimate basis. Women's bodies are different. Lots more to go wrong there, Jenny figured. Lots more not to know about.

Not that *every* woman was ignorant of how her body works. In fact, Jenny could think of one bright, shining exception, a woman who seemed to know all there was about sex, a woman who knew how to have a good time in bed, just the way men do: her mother.

Jenny's mother had been first runner-up in the Miss Illinois pageant nearly 40 years earlier. Right from the start, Jenny and her two sisters had measured their physical appearance against their mother's. How could they not? It wasn't that their mother was a vain or looks-obsessed woman; in fact, she wore little makeup, even though she was definitely an attractive woman for her age. By the time she was raising three girls, she was working as a special-ed teacher, and she clearly regarded the period in her life when she'd been a beauty pageant winner as ancient history and something of a lark.

No, it was Jenny's father for whom his wife's looks were still obviously a source of pride. Even now, decades later, Jenny could remember clearly the way her father would look at her mother across a room. Sometimes he would turn to Jenny and her sisters and say, "Girls, your mother is a total goddess. If any of you grow up to be even one-quarter the woman she is today, then you'll make some guy incredibly happy." Never mind that he himself had one of those middle-aged-guy guts and that he ate whatever was in the fridge and then some. He could look any way he wanted. But women? Women had to look like the first runner-up for Miss Illinois.

HOW SHE GOT THAT STORY

Broken: That's how Jenny saw herself. She thought her parts might not work. She thought she didn't know what she was doing in bed. She's not alone. Many women feel the same way about themselves, to one extent or another, at one time or another. You might wonder if what you're doing in bed is the "right" way to do it and sometimes you might wonder if what you've got "down there" is what it's supposed to be. Those thoughts *have* to affect your relationship with your partner. Those feelings of failure or inadequacy *have* to affect your daily life—your relationships with everyone.

Symptoms

My parts don't work right or don't work at all.

If you sometimes feel broken, then this is the heart of the matter for you. These thoughts shape your whole approach to your sexuality not only in bed but also in your mind. You believe that what you've got is inadequate. It isn't similar to what men have and it's not comparable to what other women have.

I'm not really sure how my parts are supposed to work.

The moment you begin to think this way, you're shifting the focus from your body to your brain. The problem for you then is no longer "I don't know what to do," but "I don't know what to think about what to do." What had been simply puzzling can become defeating. This sense of failure can easily become permanent: "I'll never know what to think, so what's the use of even trying?"

These may not be conscious thoughts. You may not be aware that you're hearing all these doubts, which are feeding on one another, taking you ever deeper into your isolation from your sexuality. Make no mistake: They are the perceived failings that ruin your sex life and your life beyond sex.

I usually don't—or never—masturbate.

Jenny didn't masturbate. As she once said to me, "What's the point?" If you don't know whether your parts work, or even how they should work, then why would you masturbate? It's as if what's "down there" doesn't belong to you, so you keep your distance.

I don't know how to tell my lover what to do.

If you don't know how to talk to yourself about your genitals or any other aspect of your sexuality, you certainly won't know how to talk to your lover. Even if you did try to muster the confidence and intimacy to talk to your lover about what you want in bed, you wouldn't know what to say!

I don't even think I have orgasms, or I have orgasms, but I don't think they're the kind other women have.

There's a name for the chronic failure to have orgasms: anorgasmia. A woman who lives in isolation from her sexuality can hardly be expected to experience much pleasure from sexual intimacy, let alone from the physical release. Everyone around her seems to be having orgasms! Or . . . are they? If you're one of these anorgasmic women, then you might wind up feeling isolated not only from your own sexuality but also from everyone else's. You might even begin to doubt that women even have orgasms. Maybe (you think) they're a myth. Maybe all those other women out there are faking it.

At any rate, women's orgasms are certainly not like men's orgasms.

Well, no, they're not. Men's sexual essence is unmistakably exterior. Not so a woman's orgasm, the signs of which are usually more subtle. You might see in the perceived absence of external evidence for the female orgasm not only an absence of evidence overall (hence the orgasm-as-myth line of thought) but also a sense of inferiority to men: "They've got the goods. Women don't. Or at least I don't, anyway." And so the process begins again, all the symptoms crashing together, reinforcing themselves: You don't have the parts; you don't know what the parts are; you therefore can't tell yourself, let alone your lover, what to do; maybe women don't even have orgasms; maybe men have all the luck. Think of it as a symphony of self-doubt building to a crescendo that . . . well, whatever it is crescendos do, just as long as it's not reach a climax.

I'm a total loss. Just write me off.

The feeling that there's something sexually wrong with you but that you don't know what it is can't help but affect everything that happens outside the bedroom, too. The same goes for the hunch that you're the only one in your family or social circle feeling this way. If you sometimes believe you're "broken," you might find that you're ill at ease in any social setting. You feel like damaged goods and therefore feel you can't have what others have, do what others do, or get what others get. Do you hang back in conversations, unwilling to offer an opinion? That social pattern isn't exactly a model for professional advancement, and in fact can lead to being an underachiever, as Jenny was. It can also leave you feeling the same way you do in bed: You're not good enough for the relationship you want and for the job you want.

Sources

A woman who sometimes thinks she might be broken might have been born with the same parts as any other woman, but she probably learned that they weren't good enough or good, period. She typically comes from the kind of family that doesn't name parts but instead refers to them by euphemism. This turned out to be the case with Jenny. How admiring of his wife's sexuality Jenny's father was . . . except when it came to the particulars of sex. Then it was all "you know what I mean" and "down there." Jenny's mother was complicit in this evasion, just as she was in allowing her husband to objectify her in front of her daughters. In general, by failing to name the specific parts of female sexual anatomy, parents can damage a daughter's sense of self, so that when she's all grown up she doesn't know her anus from a hole in the—well, you get the picture. Then again, maybe you don't get the picture, because you can't.

Worse, you may feel you shouldn't get the picture, you shouldn't know the parts. Otherwise, why didn't your parents tell you? In fact, a misplaced loyalty to parents can play a significant role in an adult's refusal to come to terms with her own genitals, as if to name names "down there" would be a betrayal of her parents' parenting abilities. Surely they knew what they were doing—and if they didn't, she doesn't want to know about it.

How well do you know your genitals? If you regard them as a figurative and literal mess, then you can't possibly be getting the most out of sex. If you think that the pieces are impossible to tell apart, and that they're all dirty anyway, then you might also feel that it's best to keep your distance. Taken to an extreme, this attitude can make you so distant that you isolate yourself from your own sexuality. For Jenny, this isolation was reinforced once she hit adolescence and it became apparent that the oldest of the three sisters, Sarah, had inherited their mother's beauty-pageant looks. The other two, Jenny in the middle and her younger sister, Lee, were pretty girls but not "knockouts," as their father helpfully informed them on occasion. He also sometimes took a moment—he could be extraordinarily generous with his time when this manner of paternal duty called—to encourage Jenny and Lee to lose a little weight, telling them that "baby fat" wasn't something most men appreciated. He also suggested that they might eat less chocolate and fewer french fries to keep their skin free of acne.

Jenny not only wasn't really sure of what she had "down there" but also believed that, whatever it was, it wasn't good enough. This emotional trajectory isn't at all unusual among women who think they don't know what to do in bed or that they don't have what they need to do it right. They grow up with a lack of information, and when they hit adolescence or early adulthood, they get misinformation or information they can't possibly process. They hear other girls or women discussing their genital experiences and don't know what to believe. Sometimes they don't believe what they hear, and the lesson they internalize is that all this stuff about the pleasures of sex, including orgasm, is just one big myth. When they do believe what they hear, the lesson they internalize is that their own parts are inferior. Either way, the confusion about their own sexuality becomes confusion about sexuality in general.

They eventually just give up. This surrender often happens in adolescence, but it can also happen at any other time of life. Research shows that 10 to 15 percent of women have never had an orgasm, but a woman who believes she's broken can't know that she's not alone—and not broken.

CULTURE

Everybody else seems to have parts that work. They even seem to know what to do with them. They seem to positively revel in that knowledge. They're even willing to capture their body fat and pubic hair on film stock forever!

Okay, maybe not, as Jenny conceded. Still, in that moment of self-revelation she uncovered how movies—or TV or magazines or underwear billboards in Times Square or any other aspect of pop culture—can influence our views of sexuality. Even if the occasional TV or movie character feels she's missing something in her sex life, she at least knows what it is she's missing. Not Jenny—and maybe not you, either. Maybe you sometimes feel as if you're watching the world have fun and you don't know how to join in.

That's how Jenny felt. She acknowledged as much in her descriptions of how her father sexually idolized her mother. She grew up assuming her parents had a full sex life—one that, because of her own "shortcomings," she could never hope to duplicate. Imagine what it must be like to feel that not only (as the saying goes) is life a beach, but everyone else is out there whooping it up, tossing the sexual equivalent of beach balls and Frisbees back and forth, enjoying the sensation of having their flesh energized by the surf and the sun, while you hang back in your little cabana, wrapped in scarves, afraid to venture into the light, where you know the cloud of perpetual gloom is waiting.

Maybe you don't have to imagine. . . .

WHY SHE CHANGED THAT STORY

THE TRIGGER POINT

For Jenny, the breakthrough came when she made the conscious connection between the problem in her sex life and the feeling that she was an imposter in the rest of her life. She was faking both her ability to have an orgasm and her right to sit at the same table as the other faculty members. From that point on, Jenny was able to examine more deeply how the ways she'd learned to look at herself as a child and throughout life had become embedded in her sex life and then how that sexual identity radiated outward to influence her identity overall.

Now is a good time to ask yourself if you identify with any of the symptoms or sources above. What in Jenny's experience provided a little shock of recognition for you, a sense of "I've done that" or "I've thought that" or "I've felt that"? Take that sense of recognition and look at it closely. It's the key to who you are. It will allow you to unlock the stories that have become part of your sex life and then to identify how that sexual identity has rippled outward to influence your identity overall.

SEX LIFE

If you're like most women, a problem with your sex life feels as if it's nothing special: a problem, yes, but just one more problem. Very few of the women I meet in my office walk through the door ready to talk about sex. A patient's sex life might be bothering her, and it might well be the root of her problems, but usually she'll set up her first appointment eager to talk about a particular struggle she's having with a co-worker, her children, her elderly parents, or just "life in general." (You wouldn't believe how often I hear those exact words!) Only after a few weeks of intense discussion does she mention a particularly bad lovemaking session with her partner or complain of a cumulative feeling of sexual inadequacy. That's when she can begin to see that what's dominating her life, even in the seemingly unrelated landscape of office or kitchen or nursing home, is actually a story she believes about her sexual identity. Then, gradually, she will begin to realize that this component of her life is not only important but also crucial.

It's true that we are rarely able to entirely banish the voices that give us negative messages. In some cases, these voices are as old as we are. Jenny took the early and vague messages about her own genitals, combined them with the hurtful and inaccurate messages her father gave her about herself as she grew from girl to woman, and swirled them into her own unique brew of anxiety and self-doubt. Because these self-punishing messages were in her head like some endless loop of malicious Muzak, she didn't achieve as much at her teaching job as she might have, and she never felt as if her vagina and clitoris were normal and functional, even though they were.

The fact that she had a boyfriend who loved and valued her meant little to Jenny. She was convinced Ed was just "humoring" her or, even worse, something was wrong with him, and that was the only reason he loved her so deeply. (This was a variation on Groucho Marx's line, "I could never join a club that would have me as a member.")

Jenny once told me that when she and Ed went to bed together, she often imagined that there was a giant mirror on the ceiling above the bed. It wasn't one of those mirrors you might find in a hotel in the Poconos, in which the people in the bed are turned on by the sight of their own bodies engaged in gymnastic sexual acts. Instead, the imaginary mirror just furthered Jenny's conviction that something was wrong with her. She could never close her eyes and relax when she and Ed were in bed together. It was as though she were keeping some kind of vigil.

THE RIPPLE EFFECT

A feeling that you don't "belong" in the bedroom can easily translate into the larger sense that you don't belong anywhere. You might feel a vague embarrassment that inhibits you from offering an opinion at work. A feeling of inadequacy might arise from one specific instance (a disappointing evaluation at work, for example) or from the cumulative effect of a lifetime of such incidents (a disappointing career trajectory). You might find you can barely look yourself in the eye in a *real* mirror, let alone an imaginary, unflattering one hovering over your bed.

Maybe you feel a sense of something in your life not working right or not working at all. Maybe you wonder whether there's something "wrong" with your personality or whether you can find a natural "fit" for yourself in the overall world. Maybe you feel as if you're faking it—not necessarily orgasms, but enthusiasm in bed, as well as how you see yourself in your family, among your friends, and on the job.

HOW TO CHANGE YOUR STORY

In terms of symptoms, Jenny hit the jackpot: She wasn't particularly familiar with her genitals, therefore she didn't masturbate, so she couldn't tell her boyfriend how to help her in bed. She finally came to resent the orgasmic "advantage" that men have over women. Whew! No wonder she finally felt she needed professional help.

What parts do I actually have?

Turn to Appendix A and look at the diagram of the female genitals.

Really?

Exactly. If you felt resistance to my suggestion to look at the diagram, if you experienced some queasiness, then that should tell you something right there. Your reluctance to understand your genitals isn't simply part of the problem. It *is* the problem.

Maybe you think your parts aren't enough. Maybe you think they don't work well or don't work at all. You might think your parts aren't as interesting or satisfying as a man's. How would you know? You're like someone in a man-on-the-street interview who feels free to offer an opinion about the guilt or innocence of a celebrity defendant without knowing the evidence. If you don't know your genitals, how are you ever going to learn that they can work? My advice: Get out that diagram!

Okay, okay. So how do these parts work?

Once you've learned what's what "down there" and really come to accept that what's down there isn't just one smooshy mess but instead is a collection of discrete pieces, you can begin to explore them. More to the point, take the time to explore them one part at a time. What does each part look like? As you examine it, remind yourself of what it does, what function it performs for your body. Remember: It's your body; it belongs to you.

So how can I get these parts to work for me?

Don't be shy. As long as you're exploring your genitals with your fingers, why not go "all the way"? Clear your calendar, turn off the phone, dim the lights, lie back, and go for it. If you want to use a lubricant to ease the way, why not? Give yourself over to the experience. Surrender yourself to what seems to be giving pleasure to all those other women out there. You, too, can be part of the fun. You, too, can experience the completeness, the sense of wholeness with your body that comes from a sexual release. What textures do your fingers feel? What sensations does that touching create in your genitals? What vibrations does that combination send throughout your body? If you can't bring yourself to climax the first time, don't despair. There's nothing inherently wrong with your parts. There's only something wrong with your *relationship* to your parts. If you want to change that relationship—and that's the whole point—then try again, perhaps at a later date. And again, if need be.

Don't be afraid to use a vibrator. A little wave of the Magic Wand can perform miracles.

"Wow. That was cool."

Good. At this point you might well ask yourself, what's next? Good question, but I've got another one for you: What's *more*?

Right now you've gotten yourself out of the cabana and discarded a few scarves and turned your face to the sun and dipped your toe in the water, all of which is great news. Don't stop there. Keep exploring. What feels good to you? What particular part of your anatomy feels good? Better? Best? What combination of parts feels good to touch, and better, and best?

(I have to add here, however, that if after several attempts at achieving orgasm you still can't quite do it, you may need to consult with a gynecologist, who would examine you for a physiological problem such as nerve damage. In most cases, however, the problem will turn out to be psychological. If it proves insurmountable, you may need to see a sex therapist.)

Okay, now what about him?

You've learned what works for you. You know what your parts are, where they are, what they do, and how to get more out of them sexually. Now you can share that information. You can guide your partner. You can say to your partner, for instance, that this is difficult for you to discuss and you know it might be difficult for him to discuss, too, but you have some ideas that will make your sex life better for both of you. So as not to surprise him in bed with your newfound confidence, you might want to mention these matters in advance. The crucial moment will come during lovemaking, when you'll be asking him to touch you there, no, a little bit over, that's right, a little harder, hmm, yes, hmmm. . . .

CREATING YOUR OWN
RIPPLE EFFECT

So far we've discussed only the physiological aspects of getting to know and trust and respect your body. There's a whole other side, however, to conquering your isolation from your own sexuality, and that's the psychological.

When Jenny sometimes pictured her lovemaking as if she were seeing it in a mirror on the ceiling, the effect wasn't romantic but disturbing. This is actually a fairly common psychological effect. If you can't believe you belong where you are—in bed with a lover—you might distance yourself from the scene, just as you might distance yourself from your sexuality. You observe the moment, rather than experience it.

Well, it's time to get rid of that mirror. How? Believe it or not, if you've followed the guidelines above, you're already mostly there. If you've learned about the most intimate parts of your body and how they work, if you've learned how to make yourself comfortable with them, if you've learned how to help your lover make you comfortable with them, then you're more "in the moment" sexually than you've ever been. You've claimed that part of your life. You won't need to monitor it anymore. You'll find yourself living it.

Jenny did. She worked hard at figuring out what her symptoms were and how they had developed. She learned what her distorting story was. By following the suggestions

I've outlined here, she learned how to unlearn that story. She learned to explore herself and how to guide Ed toward exploring her, too.

She learned how to look in the mirror. No, not the one over the bed. Once she had looked into the mirror as she examined her genitals, seen what her parts are and how they work, and learned for herself that they do work and that she could get them to work for her, she learned to look even more deeply at herself. By doing so, she also learned to correct her misperceptions about herself.

Once you correct misperceptions about yourself, you'll be able to do what Jenny learned to do. To look into the mirror over the sink in your bathroom, the full-length one on your closet door, the one in the dressing room at Saks. To look at yourself closely and clearly and like what you see.

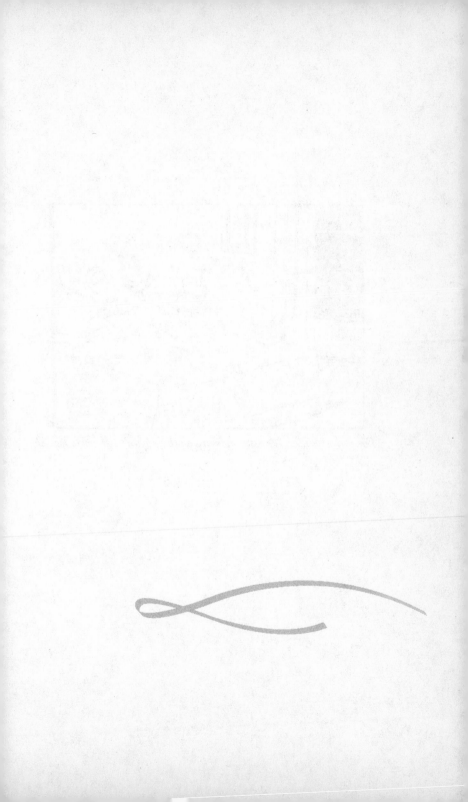

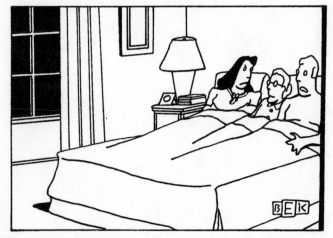

"For heaven's sake, Melissa, she's my mother. I can't tell her to leave."

CHAPTER FIVE

WHEN YOU THINK YOU DON'T DESERVE WHAT YOU HAVE

SHARON LIKED VARIETY IN HER LIFE. WHEN she moved to her condo complex, she anticipated that she would have the opportunity to meet men in a relaxed social environment, and she wasn't disappointed. To a woman like Sharon, who was physically toned and confident in her demeanor—a saleswoman for a jewelry company who had to travel and meet new people frequently—men were readily available. She had probably slept with more men than most of her friends, she figured, but each time she was interested in someone new, she was certain the vibe was good and that this relationship would be a positive one—even if all the previous ones hadn't worked out.

On her first day in the condo, Sharon met Mark in the laundry room. He was pulling his Little League coach uniform from the dryer and they got to talking. Yes, he was married and a dad; he made no attempts to hide these facts from her. His clean-cut appearance and his very openness about the facts of his life made him seem in her eyes like a real catch. Sharon knew, intellectually, that it was always a mistake to get involved with a married man and in particular a married man who lived in her apartment complex, but Mark had so many charming, unique qualities that she allowed the relationship to proceed, fantasizing that somehow it would all "work out" in the end. His marriage was shaky, he said, and she imagined that one day he would leave his wife and move across the courtyard to be with her.

The affair lasted two months. It would have gone on longer, except that one night when Mark came over after he and his family had finished dinner, the sex became very intense very quickly, and he begged Sharon to let him have sex with her without protection. He had always used a condom before, but when Sharon said she wanted him to use one now, he held her hands down and said, "Oh, come on, don't be such a baby."

"I was intimidated," she told me, "and even physically frightened—he's so much bigger than me—but I pretended it was all a big joke. The thing was, he wasn't joking. I let him do exactly what he wanted, never mind that I was being exposed to pregnancy or even HIV. In the morning, I saw him through the window taking his kids to school. He'd treated me like an object in bed and I understood that that would probably happen again. I felt empty inside, and even sort of disgusting. We broke up that day."

If Sharon learned anything from this encounter with Mark, it wasn't reflected in her subsequent behavior. Soon enough, she became involved with a handsome, older orthopedist named Keith who had a reputation in the condo complex as a ladies' man. Though he'd slept with several women Sharon knew and they had all described him as a consummate user, even "sleazy," she felt that he regarded her alone as someone special. Instead, when Keith began to break dates at the last minute and told her a couple of careless, arrogant lies about where he was going during the times when he couldn't see her, she understood that he saw her as just another conquest.

"Welcome to the club," said one of the other women she knew he'd been involved with, and Sharon had to admit that in his eyes she was just like all the others.

"Why is it so hard for me to make good judgments about men?" she wondered. She sought these relationships as a way of feeling good about herself, emotionally strong inside, like someone other people could love, yet she always ended up feeling vulnerable and used and discarded.

I encouraged Sharon to tell me about her sexual upbringing, and, not surprisingly, she needed little encouragement. She said she came from a strict Catholic background. "All-girls' school, uniforms, nuns, the whole nine yards. A rule for everything," she went on. "What you could do. What you couldn't do. Mostly what you couldn't do." She said she was in the church choir, and her mother thought she was a good girl. Sharon supposed she was. "On the outside, anyway," she added. On the inside, she said, she couldn't wait until she was old enough to have a boyfriend.

The subject of boyfriends, in fact, had been the constant topic of conversation for Sharon and her older sister, Lynn. It was the essential element in their relationship, the secret that bound them together. The two girls would lie in their beds in the room that they shared and tell each other their dreams and fantasies, swearing to each other that if either one of them became "experienced" in some way, she'd have to tell the other. The one to become "experienced" first, they knew, would probably be Lynn, two years older. The fact that her sister was willing to consider the possibility that it might be Sharon was unbelievably exciting.

The summer Sharon was 15 and Lynn was 17, everything changed. The two girls had gone out for ice cream early one evening at a nearby Friendly's. Afterward, Sharon went home while Lynn went off to visit a friend on the other side of town. Walking down a quiet street at dusk, Lynn was assaulted by a man who pulled her into an alley between buildings and forced her to perform fellatio on him.

The story of Lynn's assault shaped family dynamics for years to come. The girls' parents kept a much closer watch on their two daughters. Lynn developed an eating disorder and was briefly hospitalized a few months after the attack, though she did recover and was able, a year later, to leave home and attend college. When it was Sharon's turn to go off to college, she was relieved to be getting away from home. She assumed that in her dorm room at the state university she would not only be able to have her own active and private sex life but also be free of the trauma that had overwhelmed her life at home.

She did manage to have an active and private sex life. In fact, she fell in love.

His name was Gene, and he was a senior studying geology. She'd slept with guys at college before. Sexy, slightly dangerous-seeming men, older versions of the tough boy she'd always fantasized about in her hometown. Gene was different. His intellect was matched by a strong, lean, rock climber's body and beautiful hazel eyes. A real "catch," as her friends said. And it was Sharon, of all coeds, who had "landed" him.

"It was like he was a big fish," she told me, sighing. "And I threw him back. I gave him the old it's-not-you-it's-me routine. But this time it was true. I didn't deserve him."

HOW SHE GOT THAT STORY

Guilty until proven innocent: That's the unspoken verdict when you think you don't deserve what you have. Sharon had an active sex life, but it was also an unsatisfying one—a series of relationships that were doomed from the start and destined to leave her feeling unloved. The one time she did have a relationship that made her feel loved, she abandoned it. Like many women at one time or another or in one way or another, Sharon used sex as a way to punish herself. Judge, jury, executioner: Sharon's court was always in session but never more so than when she was in bed.

Symptoms

I like sex. A lot. And yet—

Maybe you don't. Maybe you're not willing to allow yourself the kind of satisfaction that only sex can supply. Maybe you're even willing to sabotage yourself so that you can't possibly achieve that level of completion.

Now what have I done?!

Nothing, perhaps, but that doesn't stop you if you tend to feel guilty about sex. You probably believe you've done something wrong. In time, that belief can easily become a self-fulfilling prophecy. "I'm a bad person," you might think, "so I might as well act like one."

Now what have I done . . . and done again . . . and then done some more . . . ?

If you're a woman who tends to feel guilty, you might have a lot of sex, and you might even have sex with a lot of partners (a fact that itself might lead to further feelings of guilt). Just to make you feel worse, every guy you choose might be Mr. Wrong—married, maybe, or single and just using you. If you do happen to meet a man who could possibly be Mr. Right?

Well, if what he wants is to protect you from yourself, you'll cut him off at the pass: "Let's just be friends, okay?"

Now what have I done?

Your self-destructive choices might not even stop there. Maybe you sabotage whatever you come in contact with and especially whatever means the most to you: your friendships, your family ties, your work. Anyone or anything at all, just so long as you can keep telling yourself how unworthy you are of friendship, love, success. How unworthy you are, period.

But it's not just what I do that's bad. It's what I think.

For some women, fantasies are a source of concern. If you believe on some level that a lot of what you do is "bad," you might also assume that what you think is "bad," too. Because you're a "bad" person, your thoughts might stray to the unsavory. How unsavory? For a woman who thinks she doesn't deserve pleasure, sexual imaginings often take the form of a rape fantasy. "What kind of woman wants to be raped?" she thinks. "My kind. The bad kind."

Sources

NURTURE

Sometimes the source of trouble for a woman who feels guilty isn't a real trauma, as it was for Sharon when her sister Lynn was attacked. A sexually restrictive family environment, often one relying on religious teachings, can have the same guilt-inducing effect. In Sharon's case, her sister's misfortune merely gave form to the lessons Sharon had long ago internalized. They were inevitably going to become part of her sexual life anyway, and the same would be true for just about anyone with a similar upbringing.

Short of murder, rape is about as serious a trauma as a woman can endure. In fact, it feels pretty much like being left for dead. How Sharon *thought* about her sister's trauma was a good indication she was the kind of woman who tends to feel guilty: Sharon was glad.

No, she couldn't voice this opinion to anyone. She certainly didn't voice it to me, at least at first. She didn't even allow herself to hear it. After all, hadn't she been sympathetic to her sister? Like the other members of her family, Sharon had assumed responsibility for shielding Lynn from the outside world until she was ready to try to return to her normal routine. And even then, for years afterward, Sharon always remained acutely sensitive to any signs of fragility in her sister's emotional state.

Sharon also harbored a horrible secret. It was one she kept even from herself. As Sharon and I talked, however, her secret slowly began to emerge: Where "someone normal," as she once said to me, would see in her sister a figure of sympathy, Sharon saw someone who got what she deserved.

Such a judgmental interpretation didn't come from nowhere. Like many women who feel guilty about sex, Sharon had been raised to believe that sex is something only a husband and a wife practice. Any other scenario—teen boy and teen girl, premarital, extramarital, masturbatory—would be illicit. What's illicit can often be exciting. When Sharon would lie awake at night sharing secrets with Lynn in the darkness of their bed-room, her older sister became her surrogate. Sharon's own hor-mones were beginning to rage and she was starting to entertain sexual fantasies, but because such feelings were supposed to be bad, Sharon let her sister do the "dirty" work for her. Still, she couldn't help feeling aroused on her sister's behalf. Which meant Sharon must be bad, too, which heightened the excite-ment, which heightened the sense of illicitness, and on and on. And then came her sister's trauma.

Justice was served, but for whom?

Certainly for her sister. In Sharon's mind, Lynn's punish-ment fit the crime. What about Sharon? Hadn't she, too, shamefully participated in those late-night talks? And didn't the feeling that her sister deserved punishment only compound Sharon's own "crime"? And so as Sharon matured, becoming a sexual being herself, she couldn't help harboring this convic-tion: She must be punished.

CULTURE

And so she was. Our society offers no end of reasons for women to wreak revenge on themselves for their sexuality. Again and again throughout popular culture the message is that the pro-miscuous or openly sexual woman must be punished. From the early 1930s through the mid-1960s, Hollywood even had a Production Code that made sure the "fallen woman" got pun-ished in the final reel. (Usually this meant death.) Although the Production Code is a thing of the past, the attitudes toward sexual women that it embodied and fostered are most definitely not. If you watch out for evidence that these prejudices endure, I guarantee you'll see what I mean. For better or worse (worse, I would argue), we still live in a puritanical culture. In general, society might condone bikini-clad surfers selling beer during a commercial break, or a bevy of silicone-infused blondes maximizing their cleavage on a dozen magazine covers at the nearest newsstand. Let those same sex objects become sex subjects—who have actual sex—and the rules suddenly change. For women who carry feelings of guilt, this rampant, culture-wide ambivalence toward sexuality provides all the more reason to consider themselves deserving of punishment.

WHY SHE CHANGED THAT STORY

THE TRIGGER POINT

Sharon had several "moments of truth": the affair with Mark, the Little League dad; the relationship with Keith, the ladies' man orthopedist; even opening up to me about her sister's sexual assault. I suspect the true trigger point came when she talked about Gene, the college lover. Here was a story that seemed to encapsulate everything that could be right and everything that had gone wrong in her sex life.

Is there an incident in your life that resonates in this particular way? It doesn't have to be a whole relationship; it might be just a moment in bed that you can't get out of your head.

Something that perhaps seems the opposite of how you usually behave, in the same way that Sharon's relationship with Gene seemed to stand in contrast to her usual dating patterns. When we feel we're undeserving, we have an amazing ability to build our lives in such a way that we don't get what we actually want. How we respond to the rare moment that we do get what we actually want—whether it's a relationship like Sharon's with Gene or just a moment of tenderness with a lover—can be the key to unlocking any guilty feelings we carry within ourselves.

SEX LIFE

If you're feeling guilty about sex, it's difficult to be "there"—to be present, to be in the heat of the moment—when it counts most. From your unreliable point of view, you're returning to the scene of the crime. How can you fully participate in truly satisfying sex if you think you're being bad?

Of course, being bad can be part of the thrill. It was for Sharon and for her sister Lynn when the two of them shared fantasies in the late-night darkness of a childhood bedroom. As long as you're playacting and understand that you're not in fact a bad person, then this sense of the illicit can add to the excitement in an honest and guilt-free way.

If you secretly think that you're a bad person and what you're doing is wrong, then you might easily feel that you're not worthy of sexual pleasure, that you're not worthy of this act—this *moment*. You'll . . . check out. You'll imagine yourself floating elsewhere, like a partygoer longingly eyeing the crudités while an insurance rep explains the benefits of whole life versus term insurance. This lack of presence—this emotional absence—will in turn affect the partner, who will feel that his efforts are not reciprocated. He's providing pleasure and now it's his turn, right?

Wrong. One common formula that a woman who thinks she's guilty of being bad applies to herself is: arousal, yes; orgasm, no. This turned out to be the case with Sharon. She could be like "a monkey in heat," she told me, and then a second later she would start making a shopping list in her head. For some women the no-pleasure pattern becomes so established that they might actually experience pain in order to prevent orgasm. In time a woman who feels unworthy of sexual satisfaction might prefer to just skip sex altogether. All sex, all the time, or no sex, ever: What's the difference, when neither you nor your partner is getting much satisfaction out of it?

THE RIPPLE EFFECT

That lack of satisfaction is a punishment that fits the crime, at least in the unconscious minds of some women. It's a lack of satisfaction that has taken up residence in their sex lives and now it's a lack of satisfaction that has radiated outward to inhabit every corner of their lives.

Usually a woman who thinks she doesn't deserve to have enjoyable sex wouldn't come to consult me about her problems as the result of a particular sexual incident. (Some exceptions that might prompt her to seek professional help are if the guy in a one-night stand turns out to be threatening or psychotic,

or if a sexual encounter involves a high degree of humiliation.)
She might recognize that a highly active sex life with multiple
partners is unusual, but that recognition doesn't mean that she
sees it as a problem. She might imagine herself as belonging to
the (somewhat mythical) legions of healthy women who are
screwing their brains out and loving every last minute. She
walks into my office talking about something else, something
seemingly unrelated. Her? Ha! Not a care in the world! Until,
of course, we get to talking, because the fact is, she *is* here. She
does have at least one care in the world. Something, therefore,
is wrong.

She walks into my office talking about her sex life only in
vague terms: not as one sexual act and not even as a series of
sexual acts but as a way of life. As *her* way of life, as opposed
to the (yawn!) monogamous way of life all her husband-hunting
friends covet with the intensity of heat-seeking missiles. So she
might detail her sexual experiences for me with a distinct,
almost triumphant, lack of passion.

Not that I judge my patients for the partners they're having
sex with, or with what frequency, or in what positions on which
chandeliers within the boundaries of what national historic sites.
(Okay, I draw the line at Donner Pass.) I do wonder when a cli-
ent presents her sex life to me as a triumph, because then I have
to ask: A triumph over what? Over whom? What's it to you? Why
should you care how your sex life compares to those of your
friends? What's it to me? Why are you trying to impress me?

Sharon did care. I recognized a longing in her caring and in
her need for me to care. She wanted approval . . . or disapproval.

She wanted forgiveness . . . or condemnation. Because she felt that what she was doing, everywhere, to everyone, at all times, was. . . .

"Was what?" I said to her finally, not long after she'd told me about her college boyfriend Gene and her specific sexual problem.

"Wrong," she said.

HOW TO CHANGE YOUR STORY

You certainly don't need to feel that everything you're doing is wrong in order to experience pangs of unworthiness during sex. Just a little guilt here and there will do the job just fine. For instance, do you ever think bad thoughts?

No.

Yes.

Nope.

Say it. It's true. You . . . think . . . bad . . . thoughts.

How do I know? I think bad thoughts, too. Everybody thinks bad thoughts.

What you think doesn't make you bad. It makes you human. While this is a lesson that most of us need to learn again and again, it's one that would especially benefit you if you are a woman who feels unworthy of sexual satisfaction. If you're unconsciously looking for reasons to feel bad about yourself, then thinking bad thoughts gives you a perfect excuse.

And my bad thoughts are . . .

What, exactly? I do mean exactly. I'm not suggesting that you go out and tell your friends and lovers what your deepest, darkest thoughts are. Honesty, as we all know, is not always the best policy. You can't go up to the parents of a newborn and tell them their baby is ugly. Even when honesty *is* the best policy, it can still be a tough sell. If you're someone like Sharon, you can't even go up to yourself and say, "You know what? I'm kind of glad my older sister got raped. She had it coming."

Many people don't distinguish between thinking and morality, let alone thoughts and actions. A competent therapist does, and you should be able to tell a therapist anything without fear of judgment, but that might not be an option at this point in your life—and it's certainly not an option as you're reading this page. Nonetheless, you might find the courage to open up to yourself if you compare your deepest, darkest secrets to Sharon's own extreme situation.

When Sharon secretly took satisfaction in the tragedy that befell her older sister, she wasn't being cruel or inhuman. She was responding to the powerful conflict in herself between the principles she was raised to believe about sexuality in general and the feelings she herself was experiencing about her sister's sexuality, as well as about her own. She was responding to the deep relationship between what's illicit and what's arousing. In a way, her sister's horrible misfortune freed her. It resolved those conflicts. It even reassured Sharon that her parents were right after all, that society is right, that good girls don't do certain things, and if they do, then they've got what's coming to them.

Your own secrets might not be quite as deep and dark as Sharon's. Still, chances are that from time to time you beat yourself up about "bad" thoughts. My advice is to get them out in the open. Sharon did. Over time she was able to tell me about her deeply conflicted response to her sister's rape. More important, she was able to tell herself about it. Now I'm asking you to do the same. Tell yourself which thoughts you feel worst about. Expose those thoughts to the light of day. There, I'm confident, you'll see them for what they are, just as Sharon did: thoughts, not actions. Maybe not kind thoughts; not generous thoughts; not warm and fuzzy and noble thoughts; not thoughts you'd want to confess to a friend or lover. But just . . . thoughts. Wishes. Fantasies.

Speaking of which—

Don't even ask. I don't know what my fantasies are.

Fantasies are a crucial part of everyone's sex life. If you don't believe me, ask my patients: In Appendix B I've compiled a Top 10 list of my patients' all-time favorite fantasies. Some of the fantasies might seem familiar. Others might surprise you. What they all have in common is that they're just fantasies— thoughts, not actions. Thoughts that help these women indulge their innermost desires.

If you're a woman who's already feeling a little guilty, the arrival of a fantasy might well be your cue to exit. You could still have sex, and you could even have a lot of sex, but you might not allow the pleasure of sex to reach its natural fruition. If you feel you don't deserve to have an orgasm, you might suppress it. You might mentally leave the moment and focus on something else—what to make for dinner, or that funny thing Jon Stewart said on *The Daily Show* last night. You might think about anything but sex.

That's exactly where fantasies come in. Ask yourself: Do you check out during sex? Does your mind get up and leave the bedroom, even while your body is still going through the motions? If so, when? What thoughts propel you elsewhere? That's the key; that's the moment to catch hold of. You're getting up and leaving not because you're bored or because you don't deserve pleasure. You're fleeing because something has scared you.

What? Only you can say. Whatever it is, it's (what else?) "bad." It's probably not a pleasurable fantasy or at least not a fantasy that you would like to believe is pleasurable. It's a fantasy of pain, of punishment. It's often—not always, but often—a fantasy of rape.

That's just sick.

Actually, that's just normal. Rape fantasies are probably the most common I've encountered among women in my practice. Of course, not all women who have a rape fantasy do so out of guilt. In my experience almost every woman who feels guilty about sex also has a rape fantasy.

I'm not speaking of real-life rape; I hope I've made clear by now just how horrific rape is. I'm talking about a fantasy of rape, and that's completely different.

For Sharon, these fantasies of rape actually preceded her sister's real-life rape. What happened to Lynn only ensured that Sharon would find her fantasies reprehensible, and in time she managed to pretty much convince herself that they didn't exist. With my encouragement and support, she eventually acknowledged that she'd had rape fantasies for as long as she could remember. In fact, she told me, a hint of confusion creeping into her voice, it was a rape fantasy that she could never tell her sister, back when they were sharing a bedroom and supposedly telling each other *everything*. Sharon recounted the fantasy for me now.

Occasionally she had imagined that she was lying under a tree with a tough older boy she'd seen around town. In these fantasies, he would tie her to the trunk of a tree and kiss her harshly, running his sandpaper-rough cheek against her own smooth face. When she told me what her dominant adult fantasy was, it turned out to be not much different from the fantasy she'd had as an adolescent. Sharon said that sometimes she would see her building's handyman ("He's the son of the super, and he's Hispanic, and he's *hot*," she told me), and for just a moment she would imagine what it would be like if she came home one day and found him in her apartment and he started—

Here she stopped telling me what would happen, because

here is where she had never allowed her mind to go on its own. I asked her what she thought would happen next. She lowered her eyes. She twisted a tissue in her hands. After a long, long pause, she told me: "He'd tie me to the bed, and he'd screw me really hard."

When she looked up at me her eyes were brimming. "How can I even think about being raped when my sister's been through this nightmare?" she said. "How can the idea of a man forcing himself on me even seem *hot*? Something must really be wrong with me."

I told her nothing was wrong with her and she seemed surprised and even a little relieved when I mentioned how common rape fantasies are among women. I told her that a rape fantasy is about power. It involves who gets to be in control and who doesn't. Often it allows a woman to imagine herself in both roles: the rapist and the victim, the oppressor and the oppressed.

Until that moment, however, Sharon's guilt had served as a kind of third stern parent, warning her against images that hadn't been preapproved. The fantasies that had been exciting when she was young were no longer acceptable, so she found herself facing a void. In bed with men, she was unable to follow through and respond. It was as though she was facing a blank wall instead of an interesting and compelling tapestry.

Do you find yourself confronting a blank wall during sex? If so, then ask yourself: Does a rape fantasy appeal to you?

And what if it does?

Go with it. Explore it, and not just intellectually. Physically. See if you can incorporate it into your sex life.

Instead of checking out at the moment a "bad" fantasy begins to creep into your consciousness, try checking *in*. Try letting the fantasy guide you, rather than letting you guide it. See where it goes. See where it takes you. It may be a place you like, and if it's a place you and your partner can explore together, then more power to you—and remember, power, in a rape fantasy, is the name of the game, but safety is what makes the game possible.

Power is another way of thinking about control and a rape fantasy is therefore an exercise not in danger, not in risk, but in trust—in knowing how far you can go without hurting yourself or your partner. For this reason, it's essential you and your partner agree on the boundaries. What I'm encouraging here is not sadism (though that approach to sexuality is one that many people find appealing). I'm thinking more along the lines of light bondage. One of you tying the other to a bedpost, perhaps, or one of you wearing a blindfold. Hands bound behind the back, perhaps. Whatever you and your partner work out together so that both of you are comfortable with the role-playing, and only as long as you both agree in advance that "Stop!" means stop and "No!" means no.

Yeah, but I don't just think bad things, I don't just think embarrassing fantasies.

If you're looking for reasons to feel bad about yourself, what better reason than to actually be bad? To hurt others. To hurt yourself. Maybe you've slept around or broken up marriages. Maybe you've made sure that when you wake up in the morning, you can't bear to think about what you did the night before or with whom. You can find a million ways to make sure you'll feel bad about yourself.

How can you possibly overcome everything "bad" that you've done? After all, as the saying goes, what's done is done. Yes, but a more useful question is: What precisely is it that you've done?

Before you can answer that, the first thing you need to do is get a reality check. Among women who feel really guilty, depression is not at all uncommon, and depression can serve as a scrim between the depressed person and reality—a darkening presence that distorts and obscures what's on the other side. The first thing you should ask yourself is: Are you depressed? Is your voice flat, your general manner distanced? Do you use sleep as a way to restore yourself, as most people do, or as a way to go unconscious for a while—to get away from life? If so, then you should visit a doctor. If it turns out that you're suffering from clinical depression, then you simply won't be able to trust yourself to evaluate what you've done in your life that's so wrong.

Even if you're not clinically depressed, your judgments about yourself are still questionable. That's the nature of this particular beast, isn't it? If you think you need to feel bad, then you'll take every opportunity to find evidence that you *are* bad. Ask yourself: What have you done that's so bad?

Just as saying your bad thoughts aloud, just as admitting to yourself what your bad fantasies are, so confronting your worst excesses or betrayals can be a powerful balm. So be honest. Be ruthless.

Okay. Now I feel really bad.

That's good. You don't want to go through the rest of your life feeling really bad, of course. For now, feeling really bad about what you've done isn't the worst thing. Far better that this reality be out in the open than lurking somewhere, shapeless and shadowy and vaguely understood and always, always menacing. Part of the burden of this reality being out in the open is the recognition that, just as being paranoid doesn't mean you're not being followed, feeling guilty doesn't mean you haven't done some bad things. The difference now is that at least you know who's actually following you; you know what those bad things really are.

Um, still not feeling better here, Dr. Saltz.

Okay, hold on. I'm coming to the "feeling better" part. Your "bad" thoughts are thoughts and therefore normal. Your "bad" fantasies are merely more thoughts and therefore also normal. Your bad deeds might well be bad by any social standard. That doesn't mean you can't find forgiveness for them.

In her heart of hearts, forgiveness is what a woman who feels guilty wants. Harsh judgment may be what she seeks, mostly from herself but often from others. Harsh judgment is what she gets, too. The flip side of condemnation is absolution, and this is what she also positively craves, though she might not know it.

Sharon thought her sister had it coming to her. Sharon thought she herself had it coming. From time to time you probably think you have it coming to you, too—whatever "it" might be. You cross the imaginary line in your mind separating what's acceptable from what's not, and you ask what's the use in even hoping for forgiveness. After all, there's no going back now.

There is a way to go back. "Going back" doesn't mean seeking approval from a parent who instilled disapproval in you years ago, and it doesn't mean seeking approval from a society that has instilled in you its own form of disapproval regarding sex. It doesn't even mean seeking approval from a therapist.

That's what Sharon wanted from me. Once she had admitted to being "bad" and had begun to experience the freedom that comes from unburdening the soul, every further confession she made carried that hidden plea: *Forgive me.*

She wanted me to tell her that she wasn't so bad after all. She wanted approval. She wanted absolution.

I knew that coming from me, it would be meaningless. In the backward landscape of a guilty conscience, anybody who cares about a "bad" person must be wrong, or misguided, or lame. If I offered Sharon approval, I'd just be one more nice person she'd fooled, and from that moment forward I would not be worth taking seriously.

No, she had to find forgiveness in herself.

CREATING A NEW RIPPLE EFFECT

From time to time that's what you might have to do, too: Find forgiveness in yourself. Yes, that same self that's "guilty," that keeps secrets, that wishes ill of others, that engages in self-defeating sex of one sort or another. This is the self that is, in a word, human, that behaves the way that everyone else behaves, in one way or another, at one time or another. That person is every bit as imperfect as anyone else you might encounter in bed, at work, on the street. That self is the only one that can forgive you. If you can do that—well, really now: How bad can you be?

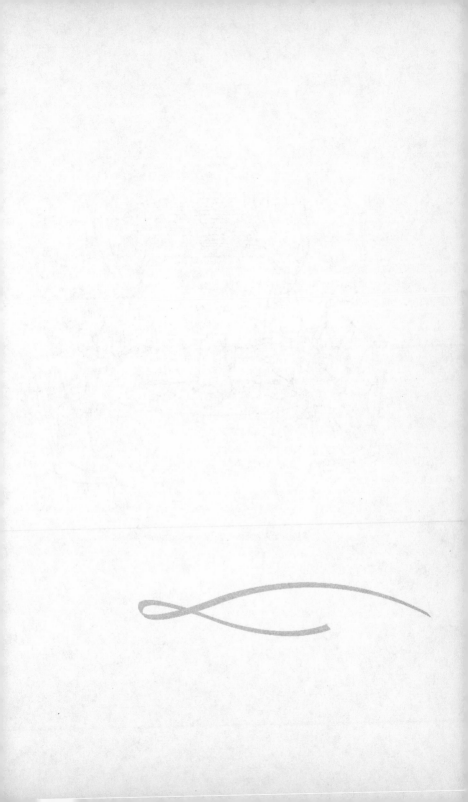

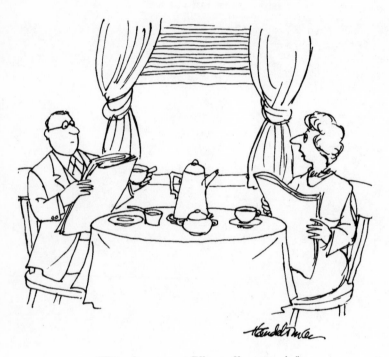

"Pass the cream or I'll cut off your penis."

CHAPTER SIX

WHEN YOU THINK YOU WANT WHAT YOU DON'T HAVE

PEGGY HAD GROWN ACCUSTOMED TO THINKING of herself as part of Peggy-and-Bob. She and her husband had one of those marriages that other people talked about. Where some relationships were secure, theirs was Gibraltar. Her entire family unit was strong, in fact, and everyone credited Peggy with this security and closeness. She was one of those mothers and wives who held everything together, who knew where the electrical tape and missing library book were, who could help a child study for an algebra test, pack delicious snacks for a hungry team of 12-year-old soccer players, and talk a nervous husband down from the emotional ledge before an important meeting at work.

Peggy had held a demanding marketing job at Revlon for many years and she had always prided herself on being good at what she did. She was definitely a "people person," someone who was comfortable speaking her mind and making others feel relaxed and open. She rose quickly at her job. After the kids were born she and Bob had sat down and discussed where they saw everything going. They didn't want to become one of those families that always seemed chaotic, so they decided that, at least for the time being, Peggy would leave her job (Bob's salary was high, and he had just gotten a promotion) and become a full-time mother in the upscale suburb where they had recently moved.

Once she left, she never looked back. Life in her town was absorbing, what with participating in her book group, taking care of the house, and raising the boys. When her older son started kindergarten, Peggy applied her capabilities and people skills to various school functions, rendering herself invaluable. According to one of the other moms in the grade, even if Peggy hadn't run for president of the parent association, she "would certainly have been drafted." Everyone knew Peggy was necessary to making everything fall into place.

For a long time it was gratifying to be so needed. For a long time it was enough, but while Peggy made inroads at the school, became a consummate soccer mom, and helped run her family's life, Bob was leaping ahead at his tech job, rewarded by his superiors verbally and then monetarily at end-of-year bonus time. One night, at a steak house in the city with Bob, his boss, and his boss's wife, Peggy, had to listen to various stories of Bob's brilliance and ingenuity. "We wish we could clone him," his boss said. "Maybe that should be the next project we undertake. Want to look into it, Bob?" Everyone laughed.

"It should have all been enough for me," Peggy later told me. "I mean, I have this fabulous husband and great kids and we live in an amazing house. No one's got a drinking problem, no one's bipolar, no one's going broke." She felt herself becoming increasingly jealous of Bob's power and influence. She and Bob briefly discussed Peggy's returning to work, yet somehow when she imagined shaking up the life she had so painstakingly set up for herself, it didn't appeal to her at all.

In bed at night with Bob, she began to dwell upon the sexual differences between them in a way she had never done before. Where she was small and fragile physically, he was big and imposing. He worked out at the gym before he left for the office. His body was solid, a mass of hard-earned muscle. Her own body felt "flimsy," as she described it, "like one of my kids' balsa-wood gliders that are always falling apart." Bob tried hard to make her sexually happy, and he was insistent upon knowing what felt good during lovemaking and what he could do to satisfy her. "Just tell me where to touch you," he whispered one night. "More to the left? Would that help?"

Peggy could only think: *Oh, more to the left, more to the right—what does it matter?* It was all the same down there. Where Bob had a big, showy penis, Peggy had vaguely defined "spaces," as she put it. It took nothing to get him excited. It didn't matter if she went more to the right or more to the left on that thing of his; whatever she did, she knew it would feel fantastic. Sometimes she suspected that he could lie in front of the draft from the air conditioner and get aroused. But Peggy?

She not only had to get in the mood and figure out what would feel good but also had to tell him how to figure out what would feel good. All the while she'd be thinking, "He's already had his orgasm; he'd probably rather just go to sleep than lie here and labor over me. Come on, parts, hurry up!"

At which point she was supposed to have her orgasm. "Ha!" is how she summarized her sentiments to me.

Sex wasn't the only arena where Peggy felt the disparity between her and her husband. Lately she felt it everywhere, she told me. When he came home from work one evening, having been rewarded for his performance on an account with an all-expenses-paid weekend at an elegant ski lodge (a weekend that Peggy would get to enjoy along with him), she was dismissive of the whole thing, telling him she'd heard that that place wasn't as nice as it used to be. "I don't know why I said it," she confessed. "It wasn't even true."

Peggy's need to diminish Bob a little, to take him down a few notches in small ways whenever she could, increased. Soon she was continually critical of him, and picked pointless little arguments, so much so that one evening at dinner her younger son said to her, "Mom, I think you need a time-out!"

Everyone laughed a little, which defused the tension, but what her son had said was true. She did need a time-out from her intensifying feelings of inadequacy and envy. She was making everyone unhappy. Even Bob, whose arousal in bed had always been a sure thing, had become colder to her at night, distant and less ardent. "What have I done?" Peggy wondered. "Why have I taken a perfect life and somehow sabotaged it?"

HOW SHE GOT THAT STORY

To some extent we all want what we haven't got: a raise, a new sofa, more free time. A desire for improvement is natural, and a desire for self-improvement is healthy. Jealousy, however, is something else. If we want what we haven't got just because we haven't got it, that's when trouble begins. If we want what we in fact can't have and will never have, that's when the situation gets truly out of control.

Symptoms

I want that.

Totally understandable.

And that.

Yes, sometimes we all go through periods of wanting more than usual.

And that. And that. And that.

It's when you stop discriminating that desire tips over into jealousy and envy—when you want something just because someone else has it.

Well, why not? Just look at it!

Not that you want blindly. A woman who thinks she wants what she hasn't got often wants nothing but the best. It's no coincidence that the best seems the best precisely because it does belong to someone else.

I don't want this.

If what the other person has is always better—and if what every other person has is always the best—then what does that say about your own possessions? That they're not worth much.

Guess I'm stuck with them.

You begin to regard your own possessions with something less than affection. This pattern might not be especially harmful to anyone but yourself if all you're coveting is possessions. But what happens when what you're coveting is something more personal? What happens when what you covet is what your loved one has?

Sources

NURTURE

When Peggy told me that she was lying in bed at night studying her husband's body and comparing it to her own, I asked about the other men in her life—her father and brother.

"It was like something out of a black-and-white sitcom," she said. "Every weekend my dad would take my little brother, Jake, on these outings. I guess now we'd say that they were 'bonding.' Back then, I just thought they were excluding me. Actually," she added, "I still think they were excluding me."

Peggy would sit in the window of the family house in Staten Island and watch as her father and Jake walked down the street together, her father's arm resting lightly on his son's shoulder. They would get into the enormous, sleek blue Buick and drive off to go camping or fishing or climbing or whatever activity they'd decided upon. "Sometimes I'd ask my dad if I could come along," Peggy said. "But his answer was always the same. No, this was a father-son thing, and maybe I should ask my mother to take me somewhere. But I knew it wouldn't be the same. I knew it wouldn't *count* in the same way."

She told me her mother was a beautiful dark-eyed woman. Men always noticed her and Peggy's father adored her. She deferred to Peggy's father, making sure she looked great when he came home from work and that she had his favorite drink in hand. Their marriage was "old-fashioned," Peggy said. "My mother and father weren't equals." When she and Bob sat down and decided how they wanted to live their life, it was her parents' model that Peggy vowed not to follow. Yes, she would leave the workplace and stay at home, but she would do so on her terms. She would do it because she chose to do it, and Bob would respect her for that decision.

"And he does," she told me. "And I do, too. I wouldn't go back and change a thing. But he gets to be out there, in the world." In a way, she was still that little girl growing up in Staten Island, staying behind while her brother got to head out for a day of adventure, "just because he had this 'thing' between his legs."

It would be easy to see a classic case of penis envy in how Peggy thought about Bob's ease at everything from earning bonuses and praise to achieving orgasm, but I don't really like using such terms, because I think they're limiting and inexact. The penis isn't the root of all envy for women. Still, it would be difficult to find a better metaphor for what women want.

CULTURE

The reason it would be difficult to find a better metaphor than the penis is that it's the major difference between the sexes. Back in the days when women could disperse an advancing army by lifting their skirts, the battle of the sexes might have embodied a radically different balance of power. Today, a little girl like Peggy who feels that her brother gets all the breaks only because he's a boy will continue to find reinforcement for that feeling as she gets older.

Peggy once told me she had no doubt that if her and Bob's earnings situation had been reversed—if she had been making more than he was and had the greater potential for advancement—then he would have been the one to stay at home while she would have been the one who continued working. She also knew that, in that case, everybody would be praising the PTA-running, soccer-scheduling dad, "as if he were a dog walking on two legs," as Peggy put it. But her? Where were her bonuses? Where was her praise? "I know he works hard," she said, "but I sometimes think he's got it easy. Like he got the better deal."

Certainly Peggy recognized and appreciated the progress that her and Bob's decision about their careers represented.

Unlike many women in her mother's generation, Peggy actually had options—including the option to leave the workplace and run the household. What she didn't have was equality. It wasn't so much a penis that she wanted but power and freedom and a sense of belonging in the world, which can be a healthy desire. It's the desire that prompted you to pick up this book and try to put its lessons to use. Wanting what you don't have can be a constructive force. Resenting what you don't have, however, can be a destructive force—for both your loved one and yourself.

WHY SHE CHANGED THAT STORY

THE TRIGGER POINT

For Peggy, what prompted her to recognize the depths of her jealousy was when her younger son told her she needed a time-out. In that moment she could see herself through her son's eyes—and Bob's eyes—and she didn't like what she saw.

What about you? Can you think of some moment from your relationship with a sexual partner where you thought, even fleetingly, "I want what he's got"?

SEX LIFE

If an envious woman were a man, you might laugh at him indulgently and say he has a "size issue," a *Whose-dick-is-bigger?* attitude toward life. She's not a man; she's a woman playing a man's game. She's a woman who tries to overcome her own sense of inadequacy by seeing other people as rivals. When this sense of powerlessness enters the bedroom—as it must, given its "penis-envying" pedigree—the attitude toward the partner can take on an undercurrent of resentment: "Okay, Mr. Penis, let's see what you've got."

In Peggy's case, she told me that she sometimes didn't feel like giving pleasure to Bob in bed. "I feel bad about it," she admitted. "I mean, he's a loving father and husband, and a good provider. Why should I deny him?"

"Why would you?" I said.

She thought for a moment. Then she said, "Because if I don't, who will?"

Peggy saw now that she wanted Bob to fail—or at least not to succeed so easily. In business or in bed, what better vindication could there be than to sabotage his success?

Do you ever feel this way about your partner? Do you feel that if he has an orgasm before you do, then he's hurried and inconsiderate? If he has an orgasm after you do, then he's self-indulgent and inconsiderate? Either way, you would be sending off a vibe of dissatisfaction that he can't help but sense (if only because you're making sure he can't possibly miss it). Meanwhile, you'd be gloating inwardly. You probably wouldn't be aware of it, but the warm glow all over will be deeply satisfying. That glow of superiority might eventually become the pleasure you associate with sex. The battle over "whose is bigger" will be won, but at what cost?

THE RIPPLE EFFECT

The story of the woman who thinks she wants what she hasn't got finds its fiercest, most poignant outlet in the bedroom. Because the story of envy is about wanting yet not getting, the problem that finally prompts her to walk into my office is, without exception (at least in my professional experience), the feeling that something's missing.

Peggy made clear what she felt was missing from her life: praise, power, and parity. She learned only gradually just how insidious an influence those otherwise admirable goals had become in her life. The problem wasn't only that she had unconsciously tried to level the playing field with Bob by withholding from him sexually and undermining him professionally. Those were only the latest manifestations of her envy, the ones that had gotten her to seek my help. Her envy had been there all along. It was what had fed her "supermom" identity. If Bob was going to get the chance to master his universe, then she was going to get the chance, too. For a while her mastery had satisfied her. She was as successful at what she did at home as Bob was in the office—or, for that matter, as she herself had been in the marketing department at Revlon. Only when she began to sense that her new position offered no "bonuses" or "promotions"—no opportunities for advancement—did her envy turn malicious and begin to threaten her relationship with her husband, because what was missing from her life wasn't just something she didn't have or couldn't have, it was what her husband had.

HOW TO CHANGE YOUR STORY

"Talk is cheap," goes the saying, but I have to disagree, and not just because I'm a therapist. Talk is what it takes to begin the process of healing. Action, of course, is essential—changes in attitude and behavior. Without action, talk *is* cheap. The problem that an envious woman is facing is one that action alone can't correct. It has to begin with a dialogue with her partner, because that's the person who has come to symbolize the great disparity in life that an envious woman is trying, miserably and without hope of eventual success, to overcome.

What I am supposed to say? "Hey, Mr. Penis"?

It's a start. The first step in addressing your envy with your partner is to admit to him that you're envious—to tell him, without necessarily coming out and saying so, that you envy his power. This approach has two benefits. The obvious one is that it gets the dialogue going. It also reinforces for you your own willingness to cede some control. You'll be telling him in so many words that you don't want his power and privileges and advantages—his mere presence—to be a threat to you. Simply by doing so, you'll be sending yourself the same essential message.

Just come out and tell him? He's going to love that.

Admitting to a partner that you consider him a rival can be tricky, to say the least. No, you probably don't want to spill everything all at once. It would be difficult for him to hear that he's a kind of enemy, and, of course, it would be difficult for you. It might be so difficult, so daunting, that you'll choose not to do it at all, which would be a terribly disappointing decision, considering how far you've gotten in this process already.

Ease into the conversation. Start by telling him only what you're comfortable telling him. Tell him you have this problem that you need to work on, and you'd like his help, and not just because it involves him. It involves both of you, and you'll both need to make an effort. You'll need to change, and he'll need to encourage and understand and support that change.

And then I tell him I envy him?

Well, yes, but perhaps a more tactful way of saying so is that, right or wrong, you feel he got the better deal, and that you think your feelings about this have gotten in the way of your relationship. It's acted as a wedge between the two of you, driving you apart in little ways and big, and now you want to get rid of that gap. You want to get close to him again.

And how can he help?

First, by understanding. Not just understanding the problem, but by understanding how hard it is for you to admit these things to yourself, let alone to come out and say them to him. You don't want him to give you a medal for it, but you would like him to appreciate the tremendous effort that's gotten you even as far as this conversation.

Second, by understanding that *you* understand you need to

make an effort, that you have a responsibility here and you're committing yourself to meeting it. Tell him that you have to learn how to like what you have, not just in the bedroom and not just with him: with everyone, all the time. Tell him that you know how to do it.

I do?

Yes, you do, because I'm about to tell you how to do it.

Make a list. In fact, make three lists. Tell your partner you'll need his help because at various points he's going to be on these lists.

The first list you can label "Real Competitions." These are the areas in your life where a desire to get ahead, to want something better, is a force for good. Maybe you want a promotion at work. Someone's going to get ahead, and someone's not, and it's reasonable for you to want that first someone to be you. On a private level, a real competition might involve your children's education or your own appearance. Just remember: The strategy in all these cases is to improve what you have, not to covet what you don't. For instance, you can focus on helping your children do better at school, rather than secretly wish they were other, more gifted children. You can concentrate on improving your own appearance, rather than trying to out-style your best friend.

The second list you can label "Imagined Competitions." These are the areas in your life where a desire to get ahead, to want something better, is *not* a force for good. For Peggy, an item on this list was Bob's boss's praise. For you, it might involve your partner's skill at calming the kids or cooking a memorable meal for a party of 12. Just as Peggy's satisfaction as a stay-at-home mom didn't depend on her husband's failure at his tech job, so your sense of worth as a mother or cook or any other kind of provider for your family, personal or professional, shouldn't depend on your partner not being able to help. The same principle extends to your friends' successes. Remember: The competition is inside your head.

The third list is one you're really going to like: "Private Competitions." Here's where you and you alone can bask in the spotlight, show off your talents, prove to the world that you do indeed possess something special. Here's where your partner can really help. Come up with some private arenas that are really important to you. Let's use the example of the partner who wows everyone with his gourmet talents, yet you know you're a good cook, too. Fine—tell him that you'd like to be in charge of the next dinner party. Feel free to admit to him as well as yourself that you want not only the pleasure that comes from showing friends a great time but also the praise. When the time comes, let yourself go. Be your best, and, just as important, enjoy being your best.

CREATING YOUR OWN RIPPLE EFFECT

Once you've compiled these three lists, tell your partner that you need his help not just now, in understanding how difficult it is for you to admit your envy to yourself, let alone to him, and not just in making lists but in reminding you. Maybe the two of you can develop a little signal to each other, a tug of the ear or a scratch of the nose—something he can use to let you know when the little green monster inside you is starting to peek through your carefully maintained façade. He can do this when you're socializing. He can do this around the house. He can even do this in bed. Maybe that's the most important place he can do it. What better way to erase any sense of rivalry on your part, to unite the two of you in a common goal, than to do the second most intimate thing you can do together in bed—share a laugh?

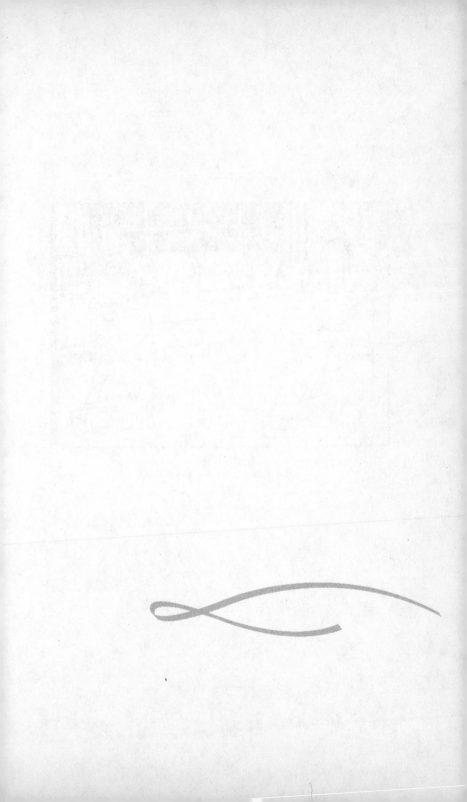

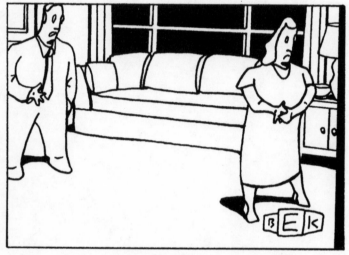

"Of course I care about how you imagined I thought you perceived I wanted you to feel."

CHAPTER SEVEN

WHEN YOU THINK YOU'RE EMOTIONALLY VULNERABLE

STEPHANIE GREW UP ON THE SOUTH SIDE of Chicago in an all-black neighborhood. Her family was big and boisterous, and she shared her home not only with her parents and four brothers and sisters but also with a grandmother and two aunts. The unofficial motto was "all family, all the time."

At age 29 she came to see me because, as she said, "I hold myself back in all areas of my life. At work I do it, and I also do it in relationships." Though she'd been dating a man named Harold for the past 6 months, she was conscious of continually withholding from him.

"Exactly what are you withholding?" I asked.

"Everything," she said with a small, rueful laugh.

As is often the case, Stephanie found it easier to talk about the work part of the problem than the relationship part, at least at first. She had been a senior editor for a publisher of travel guides for the previous 2 years. It was a prestigious, well-paid position, yet Stephanie found herself tentative and frightened whenever it came time to give a presentation in front of the other editors or to go out on any sort of professional limb. She always performed well, she quickly added. The problem wasn't the performance. It was the performing. When she got up to speak, she would have to fight against a wave of anxiety. Still, she always managed to get through the presentations, and nobody seemed to notice her trepidation. She noticed, and she worried that it was taking a professional toll. She worried that by not letting herself go, by not getting out there and giving it her all, she was keeping herself from advancing within the publishing industry. Mostly, though, she worried that her co-workers would find out a horrible truth: She didn't really know what she was doing.

It's not that Stephanie didn't know what she was doing. Maybe she did. Who knew? Not Stephanie. She forced herself to proceed through her presentations as if she did know what she was doing. What if she really wasn't up to the task? What if her co-workers figured out that this woman who had been given a good job with plenty of responsibilities was out of her depth?

It wasn't an unfamiliar feeling to her. The more Stephanie thought about it, the more she realized that it was something she'd always lived with. It was a feeling so ingrained that she hardly noticed it was there, let alone thought that she might be able to change it. It was like her dyslexia, a way of seeing words that, until it was diagnosed in sixth grade, she'd had no reason to think wasn't the way everybody saw words. Instead, she'd just assumed that she was having difficulties in school because she was, as her father told her on many occasions, "stupid."

In the middle of that large, active family, Stephanie's father was a domineering man, a factory foreman and union leader who believed that the way to keep his children and wife in order was to belittle them constantly. Her learning difficulties infuriated her father, who, while certainly not an intellectual, read a great deal and felt that a good education was essential to his children's success in life. "What are you, lazy?" he would shout as she struggled over *Charlotte's Web* as a little girl, trying to untangle the letters and words that kept rearranging themselves maddeningly, no matter how hard she worked. "No one in my family has ever been lazy about anything. Once you put your mind to it, you can do anything. And if you don't put your mind to it," he added, menacingly, "you'll do nothing, and you'll be nothing."

Although Stephanie's mother always quickly came to her defense, Stephanie couldn't miss the message: Nothing she could ever do would be good enough. Even though she understood that her father had a hot temper and was generally considered irrational by everyone in the family, Stephanie knew that she received the brunt of his anger, sarcasm, and cruel criticism, and she assumed there was a good reason for that.

No wonder she was afraid to get up and give an independent

presentation at work; no wonder she was unable to open up emotionally to the man in her life. No wonder she was unable to experience life without the need to be guarded and vigilant at all times. Her father's rage and disappointment in his daughter had left a deep, imposing thumbprint on her psyche.

Now he was gone; he'd died 2 years earlier. Stephanie had been dry-eyed at his funeral, yet inside she still suffered over his death. She recognized that she hadn't been able to resolve her ambivalent relationship with him while he was alive, and that now she never would.

I wanted to know more about her present life, but all Stephanie would say, repeatedly, was that she "withheld" a lot, and that she often felt "anxious." These were nonspecific words, the stuff of women's magazine articles, not the powerful specifics of someone's real life. Each time I tried to encourage her to be more precise about her feelings and the way they manifested themselves, I was met with similarly vague responses. Still, I felt sure that there was more to Stephanie's story. One day, out of the blue, Stephanie walked into my office, sat down, and told me.

"I guess I've been withholding from you, too, Dr. Saltz," she admitted. "As far as my work life goes, I've been pretty much up front about my problems, but when we get around to talking about Harold, I suppose I haven't been completely honest about the situation." She went on to say that when she had told me, initially, that things weren't terrific between her and Harold because she was "withholding," she really meant it in a specific way: She stops the action, right in the middle of sex. Well, not the middle, exactly. At the start. Before it gets going.

Not that they didn't have sex. Stephanie had had lots of sex. She'd been having sex since she was 17. Good sex, too. She'd had good sex with Harold; at least, she thought it was good sex at the time. How could she be sure? Maybe her idea of sex was like her idea of reading as a child or her idea of how to make a presentation at work. What if she didn't really know what she was doing, and what if Harold ever found out? How could she know she wasn't inadequate, backward, wrong?

What if she was "stupid" about sex, too?

HOW SHE GOT THAT STORY

When it comes to sex, the story that guides you when you think you're vulnerable emotionally is that you don't want it. You don't want intimacy. You don't want love. Well, that's the story, anyway. In fact, you do want love, as much as anyone else does, and as much as you do at other points in your life. To get love you also have to offer it, and to offer it is to risk not getting it in return, to risk disappointment, rejection, frustration, and pain. Better not to take that chance. Better to believe that this is simply who you are: a woman who, in extreme cases, doesn't particularly see the point of sex.

Symptoms

Who needs it?

Everybody needs sex, but if you think you're emotionally vulnerable, you don't know that. Or, actually, you do know it, but you don't really believe it. Or, actually, you do believe it, but you don't really believe it about yourself. Or, actually . . .

Okay, okay. Everybody needs sex, including me. But I just happen to be one of those people who doesn't need it all that much.

You can be guarded about sex and still like it in principle. You might understand the importance of sex for other people in theory, and you might even be able to integrate an appreciation of sex into your public life. Stephanie, for instance, exploited sex appeal every day at the office. As a publisher of travel guides, she knew how to highlight the romantic aspect of foreign settings, through photographs of a couple strolling on a Caribbean beach at sunset, for instance, or sitting in their robes on a Roman veranda and sipping espresso. The men and women in these photographs were always young and great-looking, except when they were middle-aged and great-looking. She knew what her readers wanted, and she knew how to give it to them, at least on a professional level.

Don't touch me.

On a personal level, however, Stephanie didn't "get" sex, and after a while, she didn't *have* sex, either; not often, anyway, and certainly not on any meaningful level. Because she did understand that sex seems to be important to other people, including her partner, Harold, Stephanie was occasionally willing to go through the motions, so to speak.

Does this scenario seem familiar to you? On any given night, you might sigh inwardly and surrender. That surrender is only skin-deep, literally. All you're giving to your partner is your body. On the inside, though, you've curled up into a little ball where no one can reach you, where no one can hurt you.

All right already. If you must touch me, then touch me right there, right now.

Women who tend to think they're emotionally vulnerable, like Stephanie, are often quite successful in other areas of their lives, and as a result they're used to getting what they want when they want it. For them, an act of intimacy that involves patience with a partner and mutual guidance can present a bit of a puzzle. The solution? To do what works for them elsewhere in life: They issue directives with all the authority women in their position can muster.

See? Nothing. What did I tell you?

If you're feeling guarded about sex, disappointment can become a self-fulfilling prophecy. You don't know what you want from sex, you don't expect much out of it, and then your resignation and impatience wind up not only affecting what happens in bed but also ensuring that it's a disappointment. Afterward, you can walk away from the whole irksome episode secure in the knowledge that sex isn't all it's cracked up to be. When you're feeling emotionally vulnerable, the frustration and confusion you already experience about the idea of having sex can only be compounded by the reality of having sex.

Sources

NURTURE

If you tend to feel emotionally vulnerable, the role that nurture plays in your sexual identity is usually quite specific: parental disapproval. In this respect, Stephanie's experience was extreme but typical. Her father rained criticism on her. The more I heard of her background, the more her self-protective behavior made sense.

In order to have a lasting impact, a stern upbringing doesn't need to be as tyrannical as the one Stephanie endured. Just a perpetual sense of parental disappointment can leave its mark. Disapproval as a constant downpour or as drip-drip-drip torture—either way, the destructive effect on a child's self-esteem is pretty much predictable.

The psychological damage doesn't stop there, though. Children who feel subject to criticism will not only begin to believe it must have some merit but also try to find a way to protect themselves from further criticism. They'll isolate themselves emotionally, first from the parent or parents who did all the disapproving and eventually from social interactions outside the home, just in case someone else might wound them. They'll monitor their thoughts, in case someone might find them wanting. Better to be alone, goes the thinking of a woman who tends to be guarded, than to be vulnerable.

CULTURE

This guardedness eventually can take one of two extreme forms. You know the saying "Opposites attract"? In human relations, they do so for a reason: Opposites are really just two versions of the same theme. (An old joke: "Hurt me," says the masochist. "No," says the sadist.) Women who tend to feel emotionally vulnerable often fall into two categories: those like Stephanie who strive their hardest to succeed seemingly in spite of their vulnerability and those who strive their hardest not to.

First, let's look at those who strive their hardest to succeed. You might think that if you're feeling emotionally guarded, a fear of criticism would make you shrink from public exhibitions. Not necessarily. Instead, you could overcome your fear of criticism by overcompensating. You might not do so consciously. As Stephanie once said about her adult self, sometimes she could almost hear her father's voice issuing some withering criticism, then she could almost hear herself vowing, "I'll show him." So she did.

She wasn't free of anxiety. Even an outwardly successful businesswoman like Stephanie can suffer a bad case of the jitters every time she has to stand up in front of her associates. Stephanie learned to turn this personal handicap to her professional advantage. Fearing exposure, she made sure nobody got close enough to see just how fragile she was.

That's where cultural beliefs come in. The "career woman" is a figure that even today many men and women see as somehow unfeminine. For the most part, society still finds ambition and competitiveness and aggressiveness more acceptable in men than in women, as if those qualities were sparks that could be struck only from the quartzlike hardness of the masculine form. For a guarded woman, that prejudice offers an opening. What better way to detach herself from potential emotional closeness than to become a walking, talking contradiction, an enigma, a sphinx?

I'm not suggesting that behind every successful woman stands an emotionally wounded girl. For a woman who feels emotionally vulnerable, raging success is definitely one of two directions she can go in trying to distance herself from not only her past but also her present. Even if (and, often, especially if) a career woman has a husband and children, she can still seem formidable and more than a little forbidding to her peers—conveniently so. From what I knew of Stephanie, I felt she was very likely a caring, protective mentor to many of her co-workers, their confidante as much as their boss. But such displays of sympathy and entreaties to co-workers to reveal secrets might in fact not be as altruistic as they seem; they might mask a vulnerable woman's need not to reveal her own secrets. After all, she's still the boss—the authority figure who's always a source of anxiety among employees, and even more so when she's a woman.

There's also her opposite, the guarded woman who strives

her hardest not to succeed, without realizing just how self-sabotaging she is. The conference rooms of the corporate world are full of emotionally vulnerable women suffering just as much performance anxiety, just as profound a fear of criticism, as Stephanie, yet *not* rising to the occasion, *not* overcompensating. Instead, they give awkward presentations and respond defensively to the least hint of criticism. Yet this type of guarded woman can be unconsciously responding to society's traditional view of women in the workplace just as much as someone like Stephanie is. A man who underachieves is a loser; a woman who underachieves is a woman.

Again, I'm not suggesting that a woman who underachieves is necessarily emotionally vulnerable. I'm certainly not suggesting that all women, or all men, should be competitive and aggressive. (Ambitious, however, is always fine, I think; it speaks of an effort to improve one's lot in life.) I'm only trying to explain how a guarded woman can use society's view of women in the workplace to justify a life of underachievement.

WHY SHE CHANGED THAT STORY

THE TRIGGER POINT

The day that Stephanie walked into my office and announced that she had been withholding important information from me about her sexual relationship with Harold was the day she began to recognize the true nature of her sexual identity. The pressure had finally gotten to her. She had been withholding in bed. She had been withholding at work. She had been withholding from me—and the relationship between a patient and a therapist is one that requires openness in a way that even love doesn't. A couple's sex life can survive even if one half of the couple is withholding. Therapy can't. That final pressure to open up was what finally got to Stephanie.

Do you sometimes feel that you're withholding yourself from your partner? Do you ever feel distant emotionally, even at the most intimate moments, or especially at the most intimate moments? What are you afraid of? What "secret" do you think your lover will learn about you if you open up? For someone who tends to be withholding, these questions might be difficult to answer; you would be the kind of person to withhold from yourself, too. See if you can force yourself to answer. Pretend you're sitting across from me in my office and I've just asked you what you're afraid of. Remember: Our whole therapeutic relationship depends on your ability to answer this question honestly. Once you do, you'll be able to see where these moments of sexual envy come from and how they influence your relationship with the world.

SEX LIFE

Sex is not at all a typical trigger point when a woman is feeling acute emotional vulnerability, at least as far as she knows. Consider how long it took Stephanie to talk about her sex life, even though the lack of a satisfying sex life was contributing to the vague sense of "something's missing" that increasingly was defining her life on the whole.

In this respect, society plays a role beyond defining your sexual identity on a professional level. It serves as a constant reminder of what's sexually possible but unattainable. Every sexual signal out there, every photograph of a couple strolling a Caribbean beach at sunset, reinforces the idea that something is missing. What is that something? Why are you missing it? A guarded woman has had sex, and she knows that it's not as big a deal as everyone seems to think it is, but there it is, all around her, as if it were the very pulse of civilization, yet it's barely a flutter in her life. The sense of confusion simply builds on itself, until she might not see the point in having a sex life at all.

THE RIPPLE EFFECT

If you were feeling emotionally vulnerable, you wouldn't walk into my office talking about sex. That's actually the last thing in the world you would want to talk about, and if you did suspect that the conversation with me was going to head in that direction, you probably wouldn't show up to begin with. In fact, you probably wouldn't walk into my office talking about much of anything in particular, because you wouldn't know what's bothering you. You wouldn't be guarded only from family and lovers and co-workers; you would be guarded from yourself.

Still, you would know something is bothering you. For Stephanie, it was anxiety, a common complaint among women when they're feeling emotionally vulnerable. What she experienced from time to time wasn't a genuine panic attack, which is a clinical term for an extreme condition, but it was certainly disturbing and even distressing. Even when her anxiety wasn't getting the best of her, it was still a presence, a constant reminder that something was wrong despite her seeming successes.

If you're like Stephanie, the trigger point might come not out of a specific incident but out of a growing uneasiness. Without your knowing it, the risk of emotional hurt and discovery might have become a constant presence in your life, an apprehension affecting your relationships with your colleagues, friends, family, and, most profoundly, your partner—the person with whom you should be most open. You'll certainly appear to have people in your life. Like Stephanie, you might even have a lot of people in your life, a circle of supporters who see you as a success. However, they don't *really* know you, because you don't let them get close enough. If you did, they might hurt you or discover your vulnerability for themselves.

The problem isn't that you're lonely. It's that you're alone— far more emotionally alone than anyone else realizes, and probably more emotionally alone than you yourself consciously recognize. You are alone even in a crowd of your closest friends. When this contradiction becomes impossible to ignore, when the "anxiety" it creates finally catches up with you, you'll have reached your trigger point.

HOW TO CHANGE YOUR STORY

This is going to be brief, because when it comes to strategies that the five types of women can follow in trying to change their sexual stories, the emotionally vulnerable are the exception. They simply don't have that many strategies available to them. Instead, they have one, which we'll get to in a moment. First, though, I want to ease my way into it, just as I always have to ease my way into getting past a guarded woman's considerable defenses in order to gain her confidence.

Is this going to hurt?

This is always a reasonable question when it comes to confronting emotional problems, but when you're feeling especially vulnerable, the fear of emotional pain *is* the problem. You've been deeply hurt emotionally, and you spend a good portion of your life making sure you don't get hurt again. The only honest answer to this question is "Yes."

Okay, I'm outta here.

No, wait. The only honest answer might be yes, but that's the only honest *short* answer. The full answer is "Yes, this is going to hurt, but it's going to be worth it." There are never any guarantees for a woman trying to change the story that guides her sexual identity. If this strategy works, what waits on the other side is a life free of the fear of pain that has come to inhibit your every waking moment (and no doubt more than a few sleeping moments, too).

Let's just say I'm not convinced.

Nor should you be. The strategy that can change the story of your sexual identity requires a leap of faith, but leaps of faith are precisely what you might be least prepared to make. The whole prospect of leaping no doubt sounds dubious. After all, you might fall. You might fail. Then what? You know exactly what: You'll be criticized, ostracized, humiliated. You'll be hurt all over again, old wounds will reopen, and you'll only have proved again what you already know to be true: No leaping allowed. Still. . . .

Still, what? I'm listening.

Exactly. You're listening. You're still here. If you really didn't want to consider changing your story, you wouldn't have come this far. You would have checked out long ago, right around the time that I first raised the idea that you might be guarded, but you didn't. You've proven yourself willing to listen. Now I'm asking you to also be willing to consider your options. Option, actually. One option.

I'm still listening. What option is that?

Therapy.

No.

Yes. This is it, the Big Strategy for a woman who often feels emotionally vulnerable. I mean, it's not that I couldn't suggest something less abstract—

Like what? Whatever it is, it's got to be better than spilling my guts.

Like you and your partner giving each other massages. Not massages leading to sex. Just massages. Physical contact that doesn't "go anywhere" can be a beneficial trust-building exercise for an emotionally vulnerable woman. The message of the massage would be: "Relax. Nobody's going to hurt you. Nobody's going to touch you sexually. Nobody's going to expect anything of you." (Though a little reciprocation wouldn't hurt, so there won't be any hard feelings.) Just be strict about the no-sex rule, at least until you feel you're ready. With mutual understanding between you and your partner, you can then let the next massage get sexual.

At that point, I'd definitely recommend spilling your guts.

(Sigh.)

Look, therapy is always a good idea, and of course by the time I'd be having this conversation with you in my office, you'd already be in therapy. That's half the battle. At this juncture in my ongoing dialogue with you, I would urge you to do next what I'm now going to suggest you do eventually: Ask yourself who betrayed your trust.

For a woman who thinks she's emotionally vulnerable, this might not be a question she can answer without professional guidance. After all, if you've isolated yourself emotionally even from yourself, you'll probably need an independent, objective observer to help you see where your story came from and why you're still believing it. Oh, sure, you might be able to admit, "My father could be a real [fill in your favorite expletive here]." If you're guarded, you might need professional help to uncover all the significant nuances of that story and to understand how they're still playing themselves out in your life.

CREATING YOUR OWN RIPPLE EFFECT

know that in suggesting you make a leap of faith, I'm asking a lot, but I'm not asking the impossible. I'm not saying, "Don't look before you leap." You're feeling vulnerable; of course you'll need to look. So by all means, *look*. Look back over this chapter. Look at all the details that have made you think you might be more emotionally vulnerable than you really are. Look at all the ways that your guardedness has isolated you from your friends, your loved ones, yourself.

Then, leap.

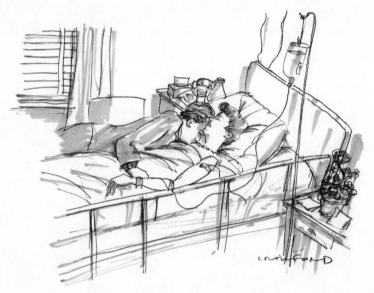

"Not tonight, hon, I have a concussion."

CHAPTER EIGHT

WHEN YOU THINK YOU'RE PHYSICALLY VULNERABLE

C OURTNEY AND MICHAEL HAD BEEN married for 3 years when she made an appointment to see me. She was a cheerful woman with a shy smile. She worked as a dental assistant and, she told me, she adored her husband. The problem, she said at first, was that she was timid. No, make that *very* timid. She'd always been on the cautious side, she said. She didn't even like being out alone after dark. Even though her apartment was only three calm, tree-lined suburban blocks from the dental clinic, if Dr. Felcher asked her to stay late for an emergency, she either arranged for Michael to pick her up in the parking lot afterward, or, if Michael wasn't available, she suggested that Dr. Felcher ask one of the other assistants. She found Dr. Felcher himself slightly intimidating, she said, even though everybody else at the clinic thought he was generally a kind and fair employer, if a bit loud. What if he turned that booming voice on her? What if he raised a hand to her? "Afraid of my own shadow, is how Michael puts it," she told me. "It's always been a bit of a joke. But now," she added, "it's no joke."

"Now?" I said.

"We want to have a baby," she said. "But it's gotten to the point where I can't even have intercourse."

I was impressed by Courtney's directness. Many women hem and haw and take side trips when talking about something that might potentially make them feel so vulnerable, but Courtney had had enough of her problem. She wanted help, she told me, and she wanted it now.

"I've known for a long time that I had this problem, but somehow Michael and I always managed to work our way around it or avoid dealing with it altogether. He's so busy with his law practice, and both of us are beat at the end of the day anyway. . . ." Her voice trailed off here, as though she'd expended all her energy on her initial burst of candor, and now she was wiped out.

Once I'd established that Courtney had been examined by a gynecologist for any possible (but unlikely) physical conditions that might have made intercourse difficult, we were able to begin looking at her problem up close, in a way that she hadn't dared do before today. Her problem had a technical name: vaginismus. Like a small but significant percentage of

the female population, Courtney was unable to have intercourse because, whenever she attempted the sex act, the outer
third of her vaginal muscles went into spasm. It was as though
her genitals interpreted the presence of a penis as a foreign and
dangerous object and quickly sent frantic messages to her
brain, telling her to do whatever it took to stop this alien
intruder from getting inside. The muscles of the vagina val-
iantly did what they could, and in short order the penis was
unable to enter the vagina. This communication between genitals and brain went undetected by Courtney. All she thought
each time she lay down in bed with Michael was that her genitals simply didn't work.

It was a suspicion she'd harbored her "whole adult life."
Whenever a man had tried to enter her, she'd felt herself stiffen
all over. She even had an image to go along with this feeling:
She was like one of Cinderella's glass slippers, into which a
stepsister was trying to squeeze a fat foot.

This problem had brought her humiliation over the years.
Sometimes her sexual partner understood. Once, though, a
young lawyer threw her out of his apartment when he realized
he was unable to penetrate her. "You're just wasting my time,"
he'd muttered as he showed her the door. On other occasions,
she simply told the man in question that she was a virgin
(which, for a long time, had been technically true, because her
hymen had not been broken during her early unsuccessful
attempts to have intercourse) and that she was waiting for the
"right someone" to come along before she had sex.

I'd noticed that Courtney had said she'd had this problem

her "whole adult life." Naturally I had to wonder how she'd regarded her sexual organs before adulthood, and Courtney was equally forthright on this topic, too.

"I always felt a little weird about my body," she said. "Well, not my entire *body*, really. I mean what's below the belt, so to speak."

Growing up as an only child, Courtney had been quite close to her mother, who had a psychological condition called agoraphobia and rarely left the house. As a result, she was usually available to her daughter. Courtney said she had fond memories of the two of them spending a lot of time together reading, knitting, going over Courtney's homework, and playing Scrabble. By contrast, Courtney's father was a big, strapping, overworked man. He found his wife's phobia exasperating, and though he often told her to get help, he himself couldn't give her any advice on how to do so. When he was home the atmosphere could be tense, Courtney told me. Between when he left for work, early in the morning, and returned home, often late in the evening, the house could seem almost sorrowful, as if his disapproval lingered behind him like a cheap aftershave. During those hours, the house was quiet, too; Courtney said some of her favorite memories were being alone in a quiet house with her mother.

The emphasis Courtney placed on that quiet was my cue. "The house during the day sounds serene in its own way," I said to her. "But I want to hear more about your father. It sounds as if when you think of him, you think of noise. Loudness. Volume."

"That's true," she said.

I asked her if any particular memories came to mind, if any stories stood out. As I'd come to expect from Courtney, she got right to the point.

The moment that came to mind first and foremost was the time she walked in on him when he was in the bathroom, and it was a frightening memory, too. She had been sitting with her mother in the den, the two of them knitting a blanket together, when she heard her father come home from work. He didn't stop in to the den to say hello to his wife and child but headed straight for the bathroom.

Courtney followed him down the hall, dragging her knitting behind her, a blanket that she wanted him to see. She thought she heard the faucet running in the bathroom, so she figured her father was just washing his hands after work. She burst into the room and saw he wasn't washing his hands at all. He was urinating—that was the sound she'd heard—and she witnessed him holding his penis in his hand and letting the urine arc into the toilet bowl. It was the first—and last—time she recalled seeing her father's penis. To her it looked enormous, powerful, a purplish horn jutting from the open fly of his trousers.

Courtney couldn't remember now how old she was, but she was old enough to know how a man's penis supposedly went inside a woman. This made no sense to her. Her father's "thing" was far too big to be put inside her mother. It would kill her if it went inside. If all penises were that big, then all women were probably in danger. Yet Courtney knew that you needed to have a man's penis enter you in order to have a baby, and right away she felt the intercourse-and-pregnancy cycle would be impossible for her.

The moment had passed in a second, but in many ways it wasn't over yet. Her father slammed the door on her, hard, but the image was already in her mind, and it never really left.

If anything, it had only grown over time. In dreams, her partially naked father would approach her, his penis exposed and far more enormous than it had been in life. It was this image of his penis that she saw as an adult, whenever she remembered that disastrous encounter in the bathroom. In adulthood, it was this image that accompanied her into the bedroom as if it were on a 60-inch flat-screen TV that she couldn't turn off. She knew she had to—at least long enough to be able to have a baby with the man she loved.

HOW SHE GOT THAT STORY

The difference between thinking you're vulnerable emotionally and thinking you're vulnerable physically is the difference between feeling guarded and feeling fearful. When you're feeling fearful, sex comes down to three little words— not, alas, "I love you," but these:

Symptoms

I just can't.

It's true. You can't. In extreme cases, you might be literally incapable of having sex, at least not without experiencing excruciating pain. Even during more moderate episodes of fearfulness, you might find the potential for physical pain so intimidating that the idea of having intercourse sounds like torture.

Well, it's true: He can hurt me.

Yes, he probably could hurt you. Men in general are stronger than women in general. That's a biological given. But *does* he actually hurt you?

Well, no. But something could go wrong. He could rip me apart.

If by "rip you apart," you mean tear your vagina or damage your sexual parts in some unspeakable fashion, the fact is: No, he can't.

Um, let me clue you in here on a couple of basic anatomical facts: Penis, big. Vagina, small.

As a rule, you're right. For this reason, it might seem that the physical logistics of sex don't make sense. This disparity in size can actually be a source of pleasure for both men and women: It can create friction that stimulates both partners. When you think that you're physically vulnerable, however, this same disparity can make intercourse intimidating and even, in time, intolerable. From the point of view of a woman like Courtney, the pertinent question regarding sex isn't "How could it be pleasurable?" but "How could it not be painful?" The parts—hers and her partner's—simply can't match, at least in her mind.

Wait a second. The problem isn't in my head. It's in my vagina.

It very well might be. That's why when Courtney complained that sex for her was painful, I asked her first whether she had seen a gynecologist for an examination. That's what I would urge any patient of mine with similar symptoms to do and what I urge you to do, too, if these symptoms sound familiar. If a gynecologist rules out a physical cause for physical discomfort, then what choice do we have but to rule *in* a psychological cause?

But it feels so . . . real.

It *is* real. Pain upon penetration; pain upon attempt to accomplish penetration; failure to initiate, let alone complete, intercourse: all real. However, what's "up there" can be as powerful a sexual organ as what's "down there." In this case, what's up there can produce a psychological cause powerful enough to actually have painful physical effects.

Like an actual spasm? A contraction?

Precisely. Psychological anxiety about sexual intercourse can manifest itself in clinically predictable physical symptoms. Not every woman who is fearful of sex experiences vaginismus, as Courtney did, but a fear of sex can sometimes manifest itself through physical pain. The unconscious of a fearful woman might not want her to have sex, so it makes sure she doesn't. The message her mind sends to her body is the one that dominates her sexual life: "I just can't."

Sources

Every person's sexuality begins to take shape at an early age, but when you feel physically vulnerable, nature can play an especially important role in how you uncover the story of your sexual identity.

NURTURE

Courtney saw her father's penis, and that was that. "Scarred for life" might be too strong a description for the effect this incident had on little Courtney's later sexual development. But from Courtney's point of view—that of a woman who sees sexuality in terms of how much pain it causes her—"scarred" might well be a pretty accurate summation of the situation. I think that in trying to understand the story shaping the inner life of the woman who feels physically vulnerable, a more accurate description might be the less inflammatory and less judgmental "influenced for life."

We can't know what Courtney was already thinking when she saw her father's penis. Nature's influence on the unconscious predates conscious memory. It's full of cues and miscues, the messages about sexuality that any infant or toddler might sponge up from her surroundings as well as from her own preliminary exploration of what the various parts of her body look and feel like. What we do know about Courtney at that moment in her life is that whatever she thought she knew—whatever suspicions or impressions she already had about the differences between what boys have and girls have—was confirmed by what she saw when she happily ran down the hallway to the bathroom door and opened it wide.

Even this confirmation might not have been enough to cause the sight of her father's penis to have such a lasting impact. In order for a message to get a grip on someone's unconscious and never let go, it must be occasionally reinforced. In Courtney's case, that reinforcement began the moment her great big father reached out his great big hand and slammed the bathroom door in her tiny little face. The message was unmistakable: "He's big. I'm small."

CULTURE

In time, this message broadened: Men are big. Women are small.

Many little girls get a glimpse of their father's penis and don't spend their adulthood cringing every time a man advances on them with that big, thick *thing* of his. Even among women who tend to feel fearful, many—actually, in my experience, most—can't trace the source of their sexual identity to such a specific and vivid incident of penis spying. Still, every woman has been influenced for life by at least the emotional equivalent of opening a bathroom door at an inopportune moment. At one time or another, we all pick up the message that men are big (and threatening) and women are small (and vulnerable), which is why so many of us do occasionally feel physically fearful.

It's certainly not difficult to find instances in which our culture reinforces this men-are-big-and-strong/women-are-small-and-weak prejudice. For Courtney, that reinforcement came in her own home, but it conformed closely to one of the most enduring and dominant stereotypes about the relationship between the sexes. Courtney's mother not only stayed home but also, because of her own fears, rarely left the house. The fact that Courtney, an only child, liked to stay home with her mother and keep her company heightened the level of identification she already felt with this role model. Courtney's father, meanwhile, came and went as he pleased. He was the one who wasn't afraid of the outside world and he was the one who ventured out there every day and "brought home the bacon." If this marital dynamic is starting to sound vaguely familiar but you can't quite place it, just think of a hairy guy in a loincloth carrying a club over his shoulder and dragging his latest kill toward a woman in a loincloth, who calmly cradles her offspring (loincloth optional) and waits by the fire.

No one knows what cavemen and cavewomen actually did, but society portrays their relationship this way because it best resembles how we like to think male-female relations work on some fundamental, species-wide level. This stereotype assumes many guises—the hero on horseback is always a man, the damsel in distress is always a woman. Personally, I think this stereotype does a disservice to women everywhere. (It does a disservice to men, too: Who could possibly live up to such advance billing?) For someone like Courtney—for any woman who occasionally thinks she's physically vulnerable during sex—this stereotype of the relationship between the sexes can only reinforce a lifelong suspicion: Men are strong. Women are weak.

WHY SHE CHANGED THAT STORY

THE TRIGGER POINT

For Courtney, the motive to get help was as simple and direct as her conversations about sex: She wanted to have a baby. Sometimes what prompts us to finally confront a problem is a slow buildup of pressure over the course of years, even decades. Sometimes it's the need to find a solution right this second—and this is especially true when the fear is physical rather than emotional. Both fears might be rooted in psychological reasons, but physical pain can be a powerful motivator to seek a solution—and fast!

Chances are that your feelings of physical vulnerability aren't as pronounced or as chronic as Courtney's, but from time to time they're probably a part of your sexual experience. Sex can and sometimes does involve involuntary physical pain, so some apprehension is natural and some caution advisable. What those moments of physical vulnerability mean to you can help you understand your sexual identity. When you feel fearful, what do you imagine happening to you? Does it remind you of anything that actually has happened to you? The answer to those questions could lead you to a deeper understanding of what role fear might play in your sex life as well as your life in general.

SEX LIFE

What brought Courtney to my door was what having a baby would first require of her. Quite often the pivotal issue in a fearful woman's sex life isn't just the possibility of pain but the impossibility of intercourse.

As compelling as pain is as an inducement to recognize the need for help, you can actually afford to live with pain if it's not a constant presence and affects only one part of your life. Even when you do feel pain, you can often stop it. Whether the pain has been a steady accompaniment to your sex life from the start or whether it's only an occasional visitor, you know you always have the options of avoiding sex altogether or interrupting the act of intercourse and asking your partner to pull out. Either way, the point isn't the pain. It's the anxiety that anticipates the pain.

That's what the constant presence in Courtney's life was— the anticipation. The anxiety. When a woman who is chronically fearful, like Courtney, first becomes sexually active, she experiences apprehension. At that point in her life she most likely can't articulate the source of the uneasiness to herself, so she'll attribute it to the jitters that anyone might feel during initial sexual encounters. This apprehension persists and only gets worse. In time, there's no mistaking it: The feeling that envelops her during foreplay is the prospect of her smallness accommodating his bigness.

At this stage, the dread need not be so specific as to involve the fear that his penis is too big for her vagina. If this pattern is familiar to you, then you might recognize this dread as a general nervousness, some uncertainty about the disparity in size and strength between the two of you overall—a woman and a man at every level of your physical beings. You don't even need to be consciously aware of the dread for it to have its effect, but the nature of the unconscious is to know what the conscious doesn't and to act on its own.

Maybe at first you feel a tightening. Totally understandable, right? Just a little anticipatory twinge. A slight spasm of the outer muscles in the vagina (technically, the outer third, but who's counting?). At this stage, sex might be a little uncomfortable but still worthwhile.

Next time, though, there's not only a general apprehension but also a memory of the twinge. What's more, the twinge was, after all, uncomfortable. What if it happens again? Your body might try to ward off that discomfort by, alas, tightening further. More discomfort. More subsequent tightening. More discomfort, more tightening, until—maybe not this evening, maybe not until an evening several days or weeks or months away, but still, when it arrives, voilà: pain!

This is precisely what a woman who thinks she's physically

vulnerable would have been expecting all along. *See?* she can now say. Sex *is* painful. How could it not be, from her point of view, what with that big penis penetrating whatever it wants? The very verb *penetrating* might be chilling: It speaks of violation, violence, and the possibility of rupture.

"Stop!"

At some point this becomes the only rational response if you think you're physically vulnerable. The pain begins to dominate your sexual life, or, more accurately, the avoidance of pain: the necessity of saying, at crucial moments during and even before intercourse, "Stop!"

Sometimes "Stop!" is a workable option. It is an unfortunate complication, perhaps, but nothing so urgent that it can't wait. As long as that's all it seems, you might avoid confronting your dominant problem or even acknowledging the existence of such a problem. In time this resistance itself becomes a problem. Consider Courtney and her desire to have a baby or several other women I've known who already had babies and interpreted the pain of childbirth as proof of physical vulnerability and weakness. If you're a woman who is afraid of having sex and you want to have a baby, the "Stop!" option becomes unworkable.

THE RIPPLE EFFECT

An unworkable option can pretty much call a halt to life as you know it. If you want to have a baby and can't because you experience pain during sex or a crippling fear of pain before sex, you're going to spend most of your time either thinking about the situation or trying not to think about the situation—trying to find something else, anything else, to distract you.

Even in less extreme cases, where the emotional stakes aren't as high, the ongoing discomfort or pain accompanying actual or attempted intercourse can complicate life outside the bedroom. It can be a vivid, potent reminder that your fears are justified— that in the battle between big and small, you can't win. Over the course of her life, Courtney had come to see shadows of her father everywhere: in the streets of her suburb after dark, in the loud but otherwise unremarkable Dr. Felcher. Her fears had finally affected how she performed on the job; an assistant rushing because she's afraid of making a mistake is an assistant who is going to make a mistake. She and I discovered that her fears had also affected her socially. Certainly she wouldn't drive by herself after dark to meet up with friends for dinner. Sometimes she even found herself making up reasons for her and Michael not to go to big family gatherings or friends' weddings. They just seemed like too much.

If you experience even some modest version of the physical fear that inhibited Courtney, then a painful experience in bed will serve as a powerful reinforcement of any other feelings of inadequacy you might already experience throughout your life. The battles inside and outside the bedroom will increase in intensity until you feel that your worst fears have been confirmed: You've lost the war.

World, big. You, nothing.

HOW TO CHANGE YOUR STORY

Not to overdo the battlefield metaphor, but in terms of which strategies to adopt, it may be useful to think of feeling physically vulnerable as part of a civil war. The two opponents are mind and matter, brain and body, "up here" and "down there"—call them what you will, but what's at stake is control of your sexual identity. Your mind is telling your genitals to shut down. Because the mind is a sexual organ at least as powerful as any other, your genitals are doing the mind's bidding—but not, presumably, without a fight.

Women's genitals aren't supposed to shut down. They're supposed to open up. They're supposed to moisten and widen and do whatever else they can to accommodate the genitals of the male sex so that the species can survive and thrive. For them not to do that, the foe must be formidable. Let's help the genitals out. Let's be on their side and help them fight back. The time has come for you to take matters into your own hands—literally.

I don't know if I like the sound of this.

Well, you wouldn't, if you feel that your genitals are sensitive to pain. But take a look at the illustration of female genitals in Appendix A. As you study that diagram, think about how pliant the parts are. *Your* parts are. The vagina isn't just this small, weak, pathetic thing, subservient to the big penis.

It's expandable. Maybe it can't quite contain multitudes, but it *is* so expandable it can accommodate the passage of a 10-pound baby. If you've ever met a man with a 10-pound penis, don't call me. Call Ripley's.

Whew. For a second there, I thought you were going to tell me to do more than just look.

I am. To know that in theory the vagina can accommodate a penis is not the same as actually seeing it welcome something the size and shape of a penis. Your partner's ministrations will always be important, but at the moment, they are only adding to the problem. Ask him to please be patient and understanding, and to leave the room, and to take his fingers with him. Prepare to explore on your own.

With what? And I mean, be specific.

Your fingers are only a beginning. The world is full of sex toys, as they're called, and some of them have been manufactured with this very problem in mind. Why not pick one up?

I. Don't. Think. So.

Yes. You. Do. You just don't know it yet.

These days we can actually choose among respectable emporiums that offer the very latest in sexual aids at affordable prices in attractive settings. So get thee to an antinunnery. Go to a shop such as Eve's Garden and you might think you're in a health food store, except them ain't cucumbers lining the aisles. What you *will* find is what Ernest Hemingway (assuming his machismo wouldn't have been threatened by what was on the shelves—an admittedly dicey proposition) might have called a clean, well-lighted place. Not unlike the local branch of the public library, in fact, and with the same slightly proselytizing sensibility at the checkout counter. I've seen clerks calmly but enthusiastically field questions such as "What batteries go with this dildo?" and "Can you recommend a lubricant?"

Wait a sec. Did you just say "I"?

"Practice what you preach" is my motto.

Okay. That helps. So I'm in this store and I'm talking to the clerk. What am I asking for?

A good first purchase is an educational film. I'm not talking about pornography. I'm talking about movies that document sexual activities as a way of, basically, showing how it's done, whatever "it" is—for instance, vaginas accommodating different shapes and sizes of penises. Yes, such films are out there, but remember that a film of this type is only a start. Seeing may be believing, but only by *doing* will you be experiencing what your body needs to experience if it's to win the war of wills with your mind.

Only by doing what?

A good second purchase is a vaginal dilator. It's an object that allows you to regulate the size of what's entering your vagina, from pinky to penis. The key is to start small, develop a familiarity and a sense of comfort with an object that size, and gradually expand the dilator. Go slowly, go comfortably, and if you become uncomfortable, *don't* go. Wait a while, then try again.

I'm still nervous.

I hate to tell people to drink, but a glass of wine can take the edge off anxiety. Just don't overdo it. Getting smashed does not preclude being anxious, and if you do find yourself smashed and blissfully free of anxiety, you could wind up internalizing the lesson that you *must* be smashed in order to have sex. (You'd also be adding a big problem to your life.)

You know, I still can't see myself going into one of these shops.

No problem. There's always mail order and the Internet.

Many perfectly respectable magazines carry ads in the back for sexual aids and educational movies, and they usually guarantee a delivery method that ensures your privacy. The Internet offers, as the Internet often does, an even greater variety of choices. If you don't know where to look, try paying a virtual visit to a venerable retailer called the Xandria Collection. The virtue of the Internet is that you can shop at leisure and in private, clicking on categories you didn't know existed and browsing through more products and descriptions than you might think the human anatomy could ever need.

CREATING YOUR OWN
RIPPLE EFFECT

I recognize that it's tempting to think in terms of a cure when you're dealing with symptoms that are physical. No symptoms, no problem, right? Well, no. If you don't address the psychological side of the situation, you'll most likely still harbor a tendency to see yourself as somewhat inadequate, vulnerable, or even destructible. Because your physical symptoms are a manifestation of what you fear, removing them is in fact half the battle. The mind wins its half of the battle by telling the genitals to shut down, but the genitals can fight back by telling the mind to shut up. If your body and its beautiful, powerful inner workings can quiet the mind long enough, you might even begin to recognize the new theme of a new story, one that will allow you to see yourself as every bit equal to a man both in and out of bed.

Men: big.

Women: big, too.

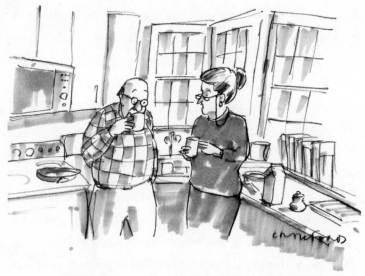

"How am I this morning? Frankly, Mister Never-Around,
I'm as horny as the middle-school band."

CHAPTER NINE

ME, MYSELF, AND I

Now, WHAT ABOUT YOU?

This question might seem odd. This whole book has been about you, hasn't it? In many ways, yes, but it's mostly been about you and your relationship to a partner. What about you, just you, and nobody else?

Not every woman has a partner, and not every woman with a partner will stay with that partner 'til death do they part. Not every woman with a partner will be having sex with that partner in a way that fulfills 100 percent of her sexual needs and desires, but every woman can, and should, have gratifying sex—sex that can, and should, involve her relationship with herself.

Young, old, menopausal, pregnant—age doesn't matter. Married, divorced, single by circumstance, or single by choice—status doesn't matter. It matters that you take the lessons you've learned throughout this book about reuniting your mind with your body and now apply them to *you*.

The advantage of working alone, at least from time to time, is that you don't have to worry about anyone but yourself. The presence of a partner can add pressures, subtle or otherwise. What's he thinking about me? What's he seeing in me? What am I thinking about and seeing in him? If you're trying to sort out your thoughts about yourself, working with a partner can be more than distracting. It can be damaging. It can rob you of the time and space you need to figure yourself out. If you work alone and you do figure yourself out, then you have new and important knowledge to take back into the relationship with your partner.

Certainly part of that knowledge is anatomical—what your parts look like and how they feel. Another part of that knowledge is what we've emphasized throughout this book: what you think about when you think about sex. Your relationship with yourself comes with the same issues, the same stories, that your relationship with a partner involves. As is the case with an intimate moment with someone else, an intimate moment with yourself can be interrupted when:

You think your parts don't work right (or you don't know how to work them).

Maybe you do in fact know what you're doing, but you just don't realize it yet. Then again, maybe you don't in fact know what you're doing—but you can always learn! Either way, curl up alone with a good visual guide (such as Appendix A of this book) and maybe a good accessory and you'll find out for yourself. Remember: Knowledge is power—in this case, the power to control your own sexuality, and with it, everything else in your life.

You think you don't deserve what you have.

Guilt and masturbation almost go hand in hand (or hand in something, anyway). That attitude is, to use a professional psychoanalytic term, hogwash. You have nothing to be ashamed of. It's your body! Do with it what you like—and if you do this right, you'll like doing it very much indeed. Besides, your body needs sexual release just like it needs exercise or a good diet or cleanliness. You have as much right to masturbate as to take a shower (or to do both at the same time).

You think you want what you don't have.

Turn those thoughts to your advantage. Instead of feeling (for instance) that your best friend's sex life must be so much better than yours because her husband is such a hunk, why not just go ahead and have sex with him? Not for real, of course—but in your fantasies while you masturbate. You won't be betraying your best friend. You won't be betraying your husband. You won't be *doing* anything except pleasing yourself. A fantasy is only a thought, not a deed, and if you can learn how to use fantasies to your advantage, they can be productive thoughts, empowering thoughts—thoughts that allow you to explore your desires and liberate your libido. (See Appendix B for a list of my patients' Top 10 fantasies.)

You think you're more emotionally vulnerable than you really are.

If you think you have trouble opening yourself up emotionally, even to the person who's closest to you, what better way to try to change your attitude than by learning to open up to yourself? Your secrets and desires and fantasies *are* you on a fundamental level. By offering them to yourself, you'll come to a better understanding of who you are, and if you can live with that knowledge, then you will find yourself more comfortable about offering it—and yourself—to others.

You think you're more physically vulnerable than you really are.

If you think you have trouble opening yourself up physically, even to the person who's closest to you, what better way to try to change your attitude than by learning to open up to yourself? Some of the fear of pain might have a basis in reality. If you're postmenopausal, for instance, you'll need to learn how to lubricate your genitals in order to overcome the natural dryness. Whatever your circumstances, real or imaginary, you can figure out for yourself that your parts are a lot stronger than you might imagine. And then you'll feel in control of an essential part of your life.

The overall point I'm trying to make about your relationship with yourself is: Use it or lose it. The vagina is a muscle, and if you don't exercise it, it will atrophy.

Set aside time for you, just you, and nobody else. Make sure there won't be any interruptions or distractions. Allow yourself to experiment. Use water, or objects, or toys, or a vibrator. Set the mood with candles, or incense, or music. Try erotica. Maybe women aren't as susceptible to visual stimulation as men, but they're responsive nonetheless—as a growing number of women are discovering for themselves, both in the service of their own fantasy lives and as part of their sexual relationship with their partners. (Of course, people can become overly reliant on pornography, even to the extent of harming a relationship, either by becoming addicted to it or by losing perspective on what to expect physically from a partner. There are terrible sectors of the pornography industry that exploit and abuse people. However, there *is* erotica for women made by women that, while still visual, has a bit of a plot and is geared toward what women find arousing.)

You don't even need to use your fingers. Many women do Kegel exercises, a series of simple physical tasks that you can perform even when you're not masturbating or having intercourse. You can, in fact, perform them whenever you want, including when you're in public. Especially when you're in public. They're a great way to make the most out of standing in line at the supermarket or driving the kids to school or sitting in your office. (Don't worry: You're not alone. The next time you find yourself in a crowd, chances are a few of the women around you are performing Kegel exercises right then and there. Really. The practice is just that common.) All you have to do is this: Contract your vaginal muscles. Relax. Repeat. How often you repeat is up to you, but the standard formula is anywhere from a couple dozen to a couple hundred times a day.

Okay, there's a little bit more to Kegels than that. You can place your hand on your stomach. You should breathe slowly and deeply. You shouldn't use muscles other than those in your pelvis. Not your stomach, or back, or legs, or buttocks. If you're not sure you're doing it right, think of what it feels like when you really want to urinate but you have nowhere to go, so you have to hold it in. (Not that you should be doing Kegel exercises while urinating!) If you're still not sure, insert a finger into your vagina and try to squeeze it. You should feel your vaginal muscles contracting around your finger, but that's really just about it.

Whatever you choose, the experience on a basic level is about the freedom to choose. You have the freedom to go in whatever direction you want, but go you must. There's simply no replacement for concrete action. With my patients I've found that I can talk and talk about their sexual identities, and we can arrive at all sorts of surprising and profound insights, but the real transformation comes when they go home and try it for themselves. I can always tell when they do. They come back to my office looking different, sounding different, and I realize then that what I'm seeing and hearing is, more than ever before, who they really are.

That's what I want for you. Only by following your inner-most desires will you be able to take the negative stories that define what you think about when you think about sex and transform them into the kind of positive stories that can change your life—that can reveal to you, and to the world, who *you* really are.

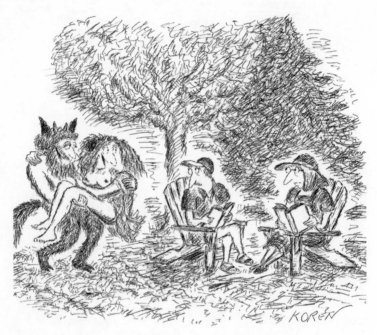

"*Our marriage is undergoing something of a renaissance.*"

CHAPTER TEN

THE NEW YOU

So now you know what your stories are . . . or not. Throughout this book we've tried to discover what you actually think about when you think about sex. I've offered five types of stories, and I've encouraged you to find yourself in them. I've identified some of the symptoms associated with each of these stories, and I've suggested strategies for changing these stories. None of this means that you've actually found your stories, let alone figured out how to change them.

If you think you have, great. You're ahead of the game. You've gotten as much out of this book as I've hoped any reader could. If you're still wondering just what your stories might be, that's fine, too. If nothing else, when you close this book and go back about your life, I want you to be able to do what my patients do when they close the door of my office and walk down Park Avenue. I want you to understand that:

- You do in fact live your sexual life according to stories.

- These stories arise from your unconscious.

- They began long ago.

- They began under circumstances that might be difficult or even painful to remember, and in ways that are a challenge to understand.

- They're still there.

- They're the stories that have taken up residence in your sexual identity and then rippled outward into every other area of your life.

- This version of reality feels real to you, but nobody who's not you would agree that it is real.

- With time, effort, strength, and conviction, you can change those stories.

- When you change those stories, you will see your sexual self in a new, more powerful way.

- When you see your sexual self in a new, more powerful way, you will experience a ripple effect throughout your life.

Like most things in life, the process can seem daunting, even impossible, before you begin. As the ancient saying goes, "A journey of a thousand miles starts with a pair of soft handcuffs."

Or not. But try something new. Start somewhere, and start right now—as in today. Start with something small, some little change that you can fit into your life with minimal fuss but as much impact as you think you can handle, or maybe a little bit more. Surprise your partner. Surprise yourself. Break an old habit. Challenge an assumption. Rock your world.

Do you make love only at night? Try it in the morning. You might be surprised. Testosterone levels for both men and women tend to be higher in the morning, meaning that the sex is likely to be more exciting. Having sex at night is one of those habits that our culture imposes on us until it feels "normal." Sex at night can certainly help relieve the pressures of the day or send us into the night with a feeling of closeness and comfort, but sex at night can also be compromised by exhaustion. If you've been arguing with your partner, both of you might have trouble letting bygones be bygones and surrendering to the moment. In the morning, though, you're fresh and rejuvenated, and last night's troubles can seem like yesterday's news.

Have you ever had sex in the kitchen? Have you ever tried to put a fantasy into practice? (Take a look at Appendix B for a list of the 10 most common and see if any of them sound familiar.) What about sex with a hint of S&M—soft handcuffs, maybe, or a feather tickler, or a sexy blindfold? As long as the consent is mutual and nobody gets hurt, S&M can be a great way to foster feelings of mutual trust. What about sex when you're menstruating? Sure, it might be messy, but it can also be a way of asserting a message to yourself and your partner that your body is working just the way a woman's body should work (and, besides, you can always clean up). How about scheduling a round of lovemaking? Our culture tells us that premeditated sex isn't romantic, but that's as much a myth as the running-in-slow-motion-with-clothes-peeling-off movie image. Many areas of your life are premeditated—work, child-rearing, meals—and they don't suffer for it. In fact, anticipation can enhance any experience, including—and maybe especially—sex. Then again, if you have trouble being spontaneous about sex, try that approach instead—complete with the clothes-peeling-off part. (The slow motion will be a bit more difficult.)

The point is, if the strategies we've discussed in this book seem like too much work or feel like they'll take forever, just do *something*. Get started in some small way and I promise the road ahead will suddenly seem like one you'll willingly walk.

Enormous emotional changes rarely happen overnight, but as anyone who's confronted difficult internal problems head-on can tell you, it's worth the wait. In these pages I've tried to help you start the conversation about the patterns that shape your sexual self. How you continue that conversation now is up to you, but I would like to make one more suggestion.

Therapy is a terrific tool, one that most of us can make good use of. A skilled therapist can help guide you through the thicket of certain areas that you might be unwilling or unable to venture into on your own. A therapist reframes the questions and comments that you bring into his or her office, letting you see what it is you're really trying to say. After all, human beings are defensive creatures. Left to our own devices, we will often do and say anything and everything to prevent ourselves from feeling discomfort. We all know that we do this physically. Unfortunately, flight is not always the best strategy. If your car is stuck in the mud, gunning the engine and trying to race out of there as fast as possible is sometimes not the best strategy. It can just dig you into a deeper rut.

The same is true with our emotions. We resist looking at the hard and unvarnished truth about ourselves, especially when we know it's less than flattering. In fact, as I've pointed out on a few occasions, that's just what our stories prevent us from doing. They keep us from seeing ourselves as others see us. In the case of therapy, the "other" seeing us is a person trained to do that seeing as lucidly as possible.

Whether you choose to make an appointment with a therapist or not, the overall goal remains the same: to change the way you think about sex.

I've referred more than once in this book to the sex organ between your ears, and I can't emphasize enough how central women's brains are to the level and quality of their sexual experiences. It sounds almost magical, but the truth is that an *awareness* of your emotional processes in all their complexity will help diminish your symptoms, no matter how long you've had them or how severe they are.

Awareness, though, is only the first step. Next comes *accep-tance*. This is who you are. Your stories—whatever they are—are the ones that so far have defined the way you think about sex, that have made you who you are. The key words there, however, are "so far." Just because this is who you are doesn't mean that this is who you have to stay. You can take that story and change it.

That's the next step: *ambition*. You have to want to change. The fact that you've picked up this book is a good sign that you want to change the way you think about sex. The fact that you've read all the way to the end is an even better sign. You're here because you want to be here—because you want to change your stories. Once you change those stories, you can join all the women we've met in this book who have taken a new story, breathed life into it, and reentered the world.

Your sexual identity, of course, is not defined only by the way you think about sex. We speak in shorthand of "the Change" to describe menopause, but there are also "the changes" (lower-case c), which are small (or more-than-small) shifts that can be triggered by anything from pregnancy to a mastectomy to meno-pause. All involve hormonal shifts that in turn will affect the circuitry of the brain. As women's bodies change, so do our roles at home and in society. Some of us go from being daugh-ters to wives and then to mothers.

Even changes to our sexual identity that might seem to have purely physical causes will also be influenced by the way we already think about sex. There are women out there who have children and yet still think of themselves as daughters first and mothers second, until sometime later in life, when they suddenly think of themselves as mothers first because of some combination of emotional and biological factors. Our own mothers' presence in our lives can affect the perception of our roles; for one of my patients, the death of her mother paved the way for her to accept herself as something other than a daughter. A young woman in her third trimester of pregnancy might feel like a ripe goddess who can control the world and everyone in it. Another pregnant woman who's ambivalent about her pregnancy might feel powerless and shackled down to the ground, a kind of female Gulliver being taken over by "little people." Similarly, an older woman experiencing the end of her menstrual cycles might suffer the loss of her own fertility. Another woman her age might enjoy the freedom from birth control and child-rearing, and end up having the wildest, freest sex she's ever had. I've met women of 70 who radiate confidence and powerful femininity, and you just know that they're satisfied sexually and in other ways. They have a great deal in common with their 20-year-old counterparts who walk down the street with a secret smile on their lips.

"What does she have that I don't have?" you might ask yourself when you see one of these women, whether she's 20 or 70. The answer is: nothing. She has the same equipment you have, no more and no less. But what she doesn't have is a story that holds her back. Instead, hers is a story that liberates her. It's an enriching story, a story of freedom and ambition and adventure, a story that features her in a heroic starring role. It's a story that ripples out into everything she does.

I often receive e-mail and letters from women who have

heard me speak on the importance of reclaiming their sexuality. They insist to me in all kinds of creative ways that the battle of incorporating a rich sex life into their routine is far too exhausting or complicated, and that in their case the lack of a deeply satisfying sex life is hardly a sacrifice. By this point I think I've heard all the brilliantly argued defenses and rationalizations. Yes, yes, you're right; it's true that women can live without fulfilling sex in their lives. Hey, people can learn to live without an arm, too. The question is: Why would you want to if you didn't have to?

Putting a voluntary end to the sexual part of your life means shutting a door on the life force itself. It means letting go of creativity and catharsis, passion and power. The cost is great, even if a woman isn't aware of it at the time. It's never too late to change. You own this amazing sex organ between your ears; it's complex and self-regenerative and filled with images. You own another one between your legs, too, and an entire body that responds to touch—that craves touch, in fact. Why should you deprive yourself, when doing so isn't abstaining merely from an indulgence, but from a world of possibility?

No one can come in and force you to embrace your sexuality. No one should even try. We are fortunate enough to live in an era and a country in which a woman can make her own sexual choices. Opting out of choosing to be sexual is, of course, itself a choice, but it's not a positive choice, merely a defensive one. Yes, there's plenty for you to be defensive about. Each day you face an onslaught of demands and pressures on your physical and emotional self. Each day you are barraged by memories from the past that you might not wish to remember. Each day you are restrained by the obscurities and the denials and the distortions that have taken up residence in your mind over the years, but each day you also have a chance to reclaim the sexuality that is rightfully yours.

I realize that I sound like a proselytizer for sex, but that's not what I'm aiming for. It's not that I think sex is an unqualified "good thing." Believe me, as a psychiatrist I've also seen the way in which sex has been responsible for damaging and even ruining people's lives.

Yes, *good* sex is a good thing. Good sex, loving sex, exciting sex, makes you feel more female, and it makes you feel more alive, which in turn affects everything you do and everyone who's important to you. Enthusiasm radiates from a sexually confident person, because the sexual confidence itself radiates, and I do mean radiates. These women *glow*.

So can you. Every day you have a chance to begin again. Today you might feel that the problem isn't in your head at all but in your genitals—that you don't know what you're doing or that your parts aren't working right. You might feel that you don't deserve the sexual identity you have, or you might feel that you want the sexual identity you don't have. Sometimes you think you're emotionally more vulnerable than you really are, and sometimes you think you're physically more vulnerable than you really are. These qualities are not only yours but also yours to change. I don't know you personally, but I do know that you desire something more for yourself than the minimum allotment of pleasure. I also know that you can get it.

Once, a long time ago, maybe long before you can even remember, you owned your own body and the world around it. The air felt cool against your skin. You had no shame and you were acquainted with pleasure. You were a baby then and everything was simple. How did everything get so complicated? You learned a story. Unlike the story of a sexually confident woman, however, yours hasn't always cast you as the hero. By recognizing your own dissatisfaction, you've got an opportunity to seize hold of the stories you tell yourself and change them. You've got an opportunity to become sexual and strong and loving and open, to become one of those women of whom people think: "Wow, she's got it going on."

You've got a chance, right this minute, right now, to change your stories, cast yourself as the hero you deserve to be, and begin to make that new you *you*.

APPENDIX A

JUST THE FACTS, MA'AM

THE ILLUSTRATED GUIDE TO YOU

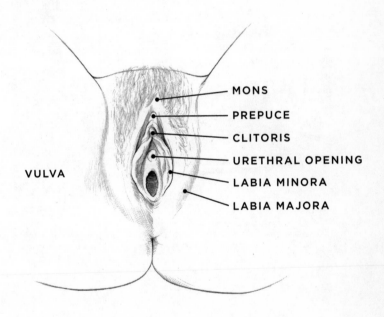

MONS

PREPUCE

CLITORIS

URETHRAL OPENING

VULVA

LABIA MINORA

LABIA MAJORA

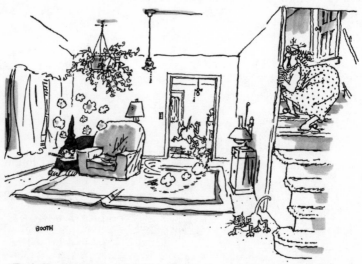

"Ready, Harold? You're the wicked troll and I'm the garden fairy, and you're very angry because you don't want me passing over your bridge on my way to Grandma's house!"

APPENDIX B

THE TOP 10 FANTASIES

I'VE COMPILED THIS LIST FROM WHAT I'VE heard in my office from women patients about their sexual fantasies. None of these are pathologic. They're *fantasies*, meaning they're thoughts not actions. These women probably aren't acting them out. Fantasies do express a wish, and I'll list below what those wishes commonly are. The *meaning* behind the wish is often more complex than just an obvious sexual pleasure. Like dreams, fantasies are personal, and what one woman's fantasy means to her is not what it would mean to anyone else, and it can sometimes be the opposite of what you might expect. For instance, the #1 fantasy can involve not what it seems—being violated—but the opposite—being in control.

A drumroll, please . . .

10. GROUP SEX. This fantasy involves more than two people having sex. It could be a ménage à trois or an outright orgy. The wish behind this fantasy might be to experience sex with members of both sexes, or to see others having sex, or to be anonymous or impersonal in the sex act.

9. SEX WITH A WOMAN. Having this fantasy does not make you a lesbian, though it may reflect an additional attraction to women (which all women have, to varying degrees—and yes, all men have an attraction to men, too). This fantasy also might reflect a desire to be cared for or to be loving toward and loved by a woman.

8. WATCHING TWO MEN. Many women are turned on by depictions of gay sex. Imagining yourself as both the bottom and the top is part of the fun.

7. DOMINATING. Cracking your whip and making him submit to you may be a reflection of wishes to be powerful and even cruel. This fantasy is common among women who have felt at some time in their lives that they have had to submit (emotionally, not sexually) to a powerful or cruel master and long to turn the tables.

6. SUBMITTING. This fantasy is the opposite side of the domination coin. In fantasies, you might assume that you're focused on playing one role, but you might unconsciously be identifying with all the roles.

5. WATCHING OTHERS (VOYEURISM). Many women imagine watching other people (in various combinations and of various sexual orientations) have sex while they get to watch. Getting to "see" the forbidden can alleviate a feeling in life that you have been kept behind closed doors and away from the action. Voyeurism allows you to participate passively and without responsibility. This fantasy also involves the pleasure of imagining being watched.

4. EXHIBITIONISM. The fantasy of displaying yourself to another or many others is often played out in ways that are not sexually obvious. Many women imagine doing a sexual performance on stage before an appreciative crowd. This is a scenario that could reflect a desire to be admired, loved, and even envied.

3. PERFORMING DIFFERENT ACTS WITH YOUR PARTNER. Many women like to imagine doing something that they just don't do. These acts could include oral sex, anal sex, a different position, S&M, and other kinds of role-playing.

2. SEX WITH A STRANGER OR CELEBRITY. Sometimes the person is a complete unknown, even literally faceless. Sometimes the person is a politician, rock star, or actor—the face on every newsstand. This fantasy might reflect a wish not only to be free of the responsibilities of a relationship, especially in the case of having sex with a stranger, but to feel important, admired, envied, or superdesirable just because of proximity to a famous person.

1. RAPE. This fantasy ranges from "He pushed me into a corner and ravaged me" to "A violent stranger broke into my house and attacked and raped me." The wish behind this fantasy might be to abdicate responsibility for wanting sex: "I didn't want to, because I'm a good girl, but he made me!" The fantasy can also suggest a wish to be passive but also to be the rapist—to be the one in control who can take what he wants and make someone bend to his will without worrying about feelings. More than any of the other Top 10 fantasies, this one, sadly, frightens the women who have it. They feel guilty and sick. What they don't understand is that this fantasy *does not* mean that they in any way really want to be raped. Instead, it involves a wish for control, power, and, sometimes, submission.

WHATEVER YOUR FANTASIES MEAN TO YOU, what's essential to remember is that they make you neither good nor bad. They just make you human.

ACKNOWLEDGMENTS

A NUMBER OF PEOPLE HAVE BEEN INSTRU-
mental in supporting the writing of this book. My husband,
Lenny, is always my most avid supporter, and I cannot express
how much it means to me in addition to how vital it has been
to any endeavors I take on. You are amazing!

Also amazing are my three daughters, Emily, Kim, and Tori,
who make every day a joyous adventure. Thank you so much,
girls, for your support and appreciation of my work and dreams.

Thank you to Richard Panek, a gifted writer, a smart and
curious man who has impressed me with his empathic ability
to stand in a patient's shoes, even when they are high-heeled.

A million thank-yous to my agent, Marly Rusoff, who has
been smart and compassionate at a difficult time in the world
of publishing. What a relief to have you on my side! And thanks
to Julie Moscow for her many insights into the manuscript.

Thank you to Shannon Welch for jumping in with both feet
and making this book both better and funnier. Also thanks to
Karen Rinaldi for having a vision of what would really be help-
ful to women and following through with it.

I am always indebted to the many women who have trusted me with their most intimate thoughts and feelings, who allow me a window into what makes us all tick, and who endlessly impress me with their courage to make difficult but satisfying change.

ABOUT THE AUTHOR

GAIL SALTZ, MD

P SYCHIATRIST, COLUMNIST, BEST-SELLING author, and television commentator Gail Saltz, MD, has been called "a voice of wisdom and insight in a world of confusion and contradictions" by Tom Brokaw. Dr. Saltz is a regular health, sex, and relationship contributor to the *Today* show, for which she hosts the weekly "On the Couch" segment as well as participates as the expert guest in a range of other related discussions. In addition, she writes a weekly "Relationship" column for MSNBC.com, is the emotional wellness expert for iVillage.com, and serves as a frequent contributor to A&E's *Biography* program. Dr. Saltz has served as a contributing editor for *Glamour* magazine and a weekly mental health contributor for the ABC/Lifetime show *Lifetime Live*. In 2004, she began hosting a series at the famed 92nd Street Y, where she interviews celebrities and extraordinary individuals about psychologically interesting issues. She has spoken with such luminaries as Woody Allen, Tom Brokaw, Katie Couric, Jane Pauley, Gail Sheehy, and Rosie O'Donnell, among others.

Gaining a reputation as the go-to person on a variety of psychological issues, especially those pertaining to women's emotional well-being, Dr. Saltz has appeared repeatedly on *The Oprah Winfrey Show, Dateline,* CBS News and *the Early Show,* Fox News, CNN, *Larry King Live,* and *Anderson Cooper 360,* among others. She has been featured or quoted in the Associated Press, *Newsweek, Harper's Bazaar, Redbook, Woman's World, Town & Country, New York* magazine, the *New York Times,* the *New York Daily News,* the *New York Post,* the *Los Angeles Times,* and WebMD.

In addition to her latest book, *The Anatomy of a Secret Life,* Dr. Saltz is the author of the critically acclaimed *Becoming Real: Defeating the Stories We Tell Ourselves That Hold Us Back* and two children's books: *Amazing You! Getting Smart About Your Private Parts,* and *Changing You! A Guide to Body Changes and Sexuality,* which was a *New York Times* bestseller.

An associate professor of psychiatry at New York Presbyterian Hospital/Weill Cornell Medical College and an affiliate of the New York Psychoanalytic Institute, Dr. Saltz has a private practice on the Upper East Side of Manhattan. She lives in New York with her husband and three daughters.

For more information, visit Dr. Saltz's Web site: **www.drgailsaltz.com.**

INDEX

Boldface references indicate illustrations.